Haematology at a Glance

Atul B. Mehta

MA, MD, FRCP, FRCPath
Royal Free and University College School of Medicine
Royal Free Hospital
London

A. Victor Hoffbrand

MA, DM, FRCP, FRCPath, FRCP (Edin), DSc F. Med. Sci.
Royal Free and University College School of Medicine
Royal Free Hospital
London

Third edition

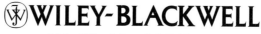

WILEY-BLACKWELL

A John Wiley & Sons, Ltd., Publication

This edition first published 2009, © 2009 by Atul B. Mehta and A. Victor Hoffbrand
Previous editions: 2000, 2005

Blackwell Publishing was acquired by John Wiley & Sons in February 2007. Blackwell's publishing program has been merged with Wiley's global Scientific, Technical and Medical business to form Wiley-Blackwell.

Registered office: John Wiley & Sons Ltd, The Atrium, Southern Gate, Chichester, West Sussex, PO19 8SQ, UK

Editorial offices: 9600 Garsington Road, Oxford, OX4 2DQ, UK

The Atrium, Southern Gate, Chichester, West Sussex, PO19 8SQ, UK

111 River Street, Hoboken, NJ 07030-5774, USA

For details of our global editorial offices, for customer services and for information about how to apply for permission to reuse the copyright material in this book please see our website at www.wiley.com/wiley-blackwell

The right of the author to be identified as the author of this work has been asserted in accordance with the Copyright, Designs and Patents Act 1988.

Wiley also publishes its books in a variety of electronic formats. Some content that appears in print may not be available in electronic books.

Designations used by companies to distinguish their products are often claimed as trademarks. All brand names and product names used in this book are trade names, service marks, trademarks or registered trademarks of their respective owners. The publisher is not associated with any product or vendor mentioned in this book. This publication is designed to provide accurate and authoritative information in regard to the subject matter covered. It is sold on the understanding that the publisher is not engaged in rendering professional services. If professional advice or other expert assistance is required, the services of a competent professional should be sought.

Library of Congress Cataloging-in-Publication Data

Mehta, Atul B.

Haematology at a glance / Atul B. Mehta, A. Victor Hoffbrand. – 3rd ed.

   p.; cm.

Includes bibliographical references and index.

ISBN 978-1-4051-7970-6

1. Hematology–Handbooks, manuals, etc.   2. Blood–Diseases–Handbooks, manuals, etc. I. Hoffbrand, A. V. II. Title.

[DNLM: 1. Hematologic Diseases.   2. Blood Cells–cytology.   WH 120 M498h 2009]

RB145.M395 2009

616.1′5–dc22   2008042564

ISBN: 978-1-4051-7970-6

A catalogue record for this book is available from the British Library.

Set in 9.5/12 pt Times by Aptara® Inc., New Delhi, India
Printed in Singapore by Ho Printing Singapore Pte Ltd

2   2010

Contents

Preface to the third edition

The popularity of this book, in both its English and foreign translations, and the rapid changes in the practices of haematology have encouraged us to write this third edition as soon as 4 years after the second edition appeared. Preparing this new edition has enabled us to improve and simplify the layout of the text and figures throughout. Also, the sections on the lymphomas and myeloproliferative diseases, where substantial new knowledge has recently been gained, have been expanded. This also reflects the frequency of these conditions in clinical practice. PET scans, which are now widely used in diagnosis and follow-up of the lymphomas, are given a wider coverage. A glossary has been added in line with other *at a Glance* books in this series and new case histories, questions and self-assessment have been added.

We are grateful to our publishers Wiley-Blackwell, and particularly Karen Moore, for support, encouragement and expert help with the preparation of this third edition and to Ms June Elliott for her expert and unstinting secretarial assistance.

Atul Mehta
Victor Hoffbrand

Preface to the first edition

With the ever-increasing complexity of the medical undergraduate curriculum, we feel that there is a need for a concise introduction to clinical and laboratory haematology for medical students. The *at a Glance* format has allowed us to divide the subject into easily digestible slices or bytes of information.

We have tried to emphasize the importance of basic scientific and clinical mechanisms, and common diseases as opposed to rare syndromes. The clinical features and laboratory findings are summarized and illustrated; treatment is briefly outlined.

This book is intended for medical students, but will be useful to anyone who needs a concise and up-to-date introduction to haematology, for example nurses, medical laboratory scientists and those in professions supplementary to medicine.

We particularly thank June Elliott, who has patiently word-processed the manuscript through many revisions, and Jonathan Rowley and his colleagues at Blackwell Science.

Atul Mehta
Victor Hoffbrand
January 2000

1 Haemopoiesis: physiology and pathology

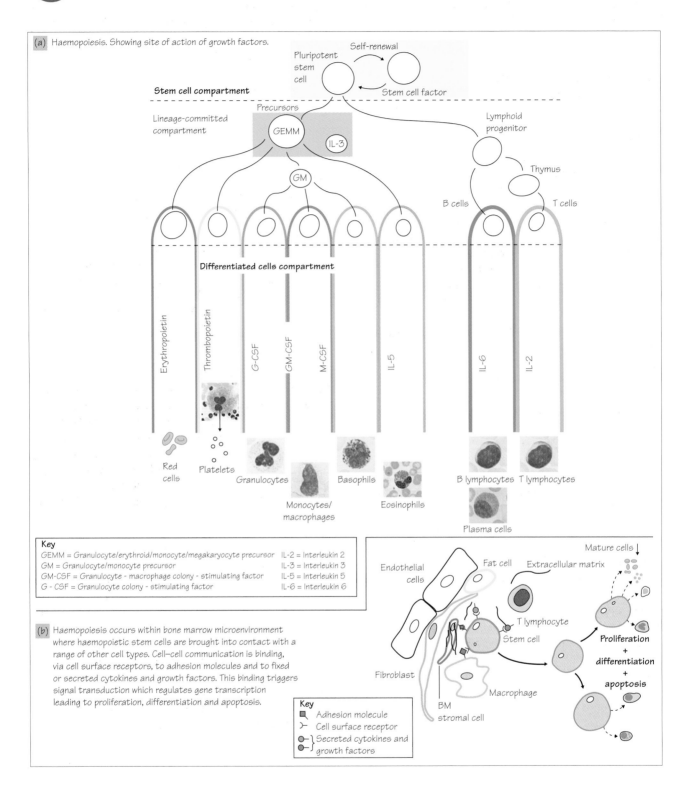

(a) Haemopoiesis. Showing site of action of growth factors.

Key
GEMM = Granulocyte/erythroid/monocyte/megakaryocyte precursor
GM = Granulocyte/monocyte precursor
GM-CSF = Granulocyte - macrophage colony - stimulating factor
G - CSF = Granulocyte colony - stimulating factor
IL-2 = Interleukin 2
IL-3 = Interleukin 3
IL-5 = Interleukin 5
IL-6 = Interleukin 6

(b) Haemopoiesis occurs within bone marrow microenvironment where haemopoietic stem cells are brought into contact with a range of other cell types. Cell–cell communication is binding, via cell surface receptors, to adhesion molecules and to fixed or secreted cytokines and growth factors. This binding triggers signal transduction which regulates gene transcription leading to proliferation, differentiation and apoptosis.

Key
■ Adhesion molecule
⊱ Cell surface receptor
●⊱ Secreted cytokines and growth factors

Definition and sites

Haemopoiesis is the process whereby blood cells are made (Fig. 1a). The yolk sac, and later the liver and spleen, is important in foetal life, but after birth normal haemopoiesis is restricted to the bone marrow. Infants have haemopoietic marrow in all bones, but in adults it is in the central skeleton and proximal ends of long bones (normal fat to haemopoietic tissue ratio of about 50:50) (Fig. 8b). Expansion of haemopoiesis down the long bones may occur in malignancy, e.g. in leukaemias, or when there is increased demand, e.g. chronic haemolytic anaemias.

8 *Haematology at a Glance*, 3e. By A. Mehta and V. Hoffbrand. Published 2009 by Blackwell Publishing. ISBN 978-1-4051-7970-6.

The liver and spleen can resume extramedullary haemopoiesis when there is marrow replacement, e.g. in myelofibrosis, or excessive demand, e.g. in severe haemolytic anaemias such as thalassaemia major.

Stem cell and progenitor cells

Haemopoiesis involves the complex physiological processes of proliferation, differentiation and apoptosis (programmed cell death). The bone marrow produces more than a million red cells per second in addition to similar numbers of white cells and platelets. This capacity can be increased in response to increased demand and in malignancy. A common primitive stem cell in the marrow has the capacity to self-replicate and to give rise to increasingly specialized progenitor cells which, after many (13–16) cell divisions within the marrow, form the mature cells (red cells, granulocytes, monocytes, platelets and lymphocytes) of the peripheral blood (Fig. 1a). The earliest recognizable red cell precursor is a pronormoblast, and for granulocytes or monocytes, a myeloblast. An early lineage division is between lymphoid and myeloid cells. Stem and progenitor cells cannot be recognized morphologically; they resemble lymphocytes. Progenitor cells can be detected by in vitro assays in which they form colonies (e.g. colony-forming units for granulocytes and monocytes, CFU-GM, or for red cells, BFU-E and CFU-E). Stem and progenitor cells also circulate in the peripheral blood and can be harvested for use in stem cell transplantation.

The stromal cells of the marrow (fibroblasts, endothelial cells, macrophages, fat cells) have adhesion molecules which react with corresponding ligands on the stem cells to maintain their viability and to correctly localize them. The haemopoietic stem cells may be 'plastic', i.e. capable of forming cells of other tissues, e.g. liver, heart, nervous system, but this is controversial. The marrow also contains mesenchymal stem cells that can form cartilage, fibrous tissue, bone and endothelial cells.

Growth factors

Haemopoiesis is regulated by growth factors (GFs) (Table 1.1) which usually act in synergy. These are glycoproteins produced by stromal cells, T lymphocytes, the liver and, for erythropoietin, the kidney. While some GFs act mainly on receptors on primitive cells, others act on later cells already committed to a particular lineage. GFs also affect the function of mature cells. GFs inhibit apoptosis (programmed cell death) of their target cells. GFs in clinical use include erythropoietin, granulocyte colony-stimulating factor (G-CSF), and recently analogues of thrombopoietin.

Table 1.1 Haemopoietic growth factors

Act on stromal cells
  IL-1 (stimulate production of GM-CSF, G-CSF, M-CSF, IL-6)
  TNF

Act on pluripotential cells
  Stem cell factor

Act on early multipotential cells
  IL-3
  IL-4
  IL-6
  GM-CSF

Act on committed progenitor cells*
  G-CSF
  M-CSF
  IL-5 (eosinophil CSF)
  Erythropoietin
  Thrombopoietin

G-CSF, granulocyte colony-stimulating factor; GM-CSF, granulocyte-macrophage colony-stimulating factor; IL, interleukin; M-CSF, monocyte colony stimulating factor
*These growth factors (especially G-CSF and thrombopoietin) also act on earlier cells

Signal transduction

The binding of a GF with its surface receptor on the haemopoietic cell activates by phosphorylation, a complex series of biochemical reactions by which a message is transmitted to the nucleus (Fig. 1b). The signal activates transcription factors, which in turn activate or inhibit gene transcription. The signal may activate pathways, which cause the cell to enter cell cycle (replicate), differentiate, maintain viability (inhibition of apoptosis) or increase functional activity (e.g. enhancement of bacterial cell killing by neutrophils).

Assessment of haemopoiesis

Haemopoiesis can be assessed clinically by performing a full blood count (see Appendix II). Bone marrow aspiration also allows assessment of the later stages of maturation of haemopoietic cells (Fig. 8c; see Chapter 7 for indications). Trephine biopsy (Fig. 8b) provides a core of bone and bone marrow to show architecture. Reticulocytes are young red cells and reticulated platelets are young platelets. Assessment of their numbers can be performed by automated cell counters and will give an approximation of the age of the blood cell population. As a general rule, the action of GFs increases the number of young cells, in response to demand.

(a) Normal adult haemoglobin contains four globin (polypeptide) chains (α_1, α_2, β_1, β_2), each with its own haem molecule. These chains undergo conformational change and move with respect to each other when binding O_2 and CO_2. 2,3-Diphosphoglycerate (2,3-DPG) binds between the β chains to reduce affinity for O_2 and allow O_2 release to the tissues.

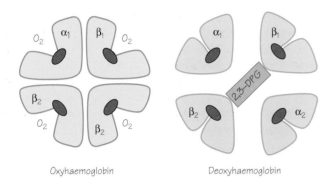

Oxyhaemoglobin   Deoxyhaemoglobin

(b) The globin genes are located on chromosomes 16 (ζ, α) and 11 (ϵ, γ, δ, β). A 5' locus control region (LCR) is important in regulating γ and β globin gene expression. Different genes are transcribed during pre- and postnatal life, and the chains are synthesized independently and then combine to produce the different haemoglobins. The γ genes differ to produce either a glutamic acid ($G\gamma$) or alanine ($A\gamma$) residue at position 136. Whereas haemopoiesis occurs in yolk sac, liver and spleen prenatally, it is confined to marrow postnatally.

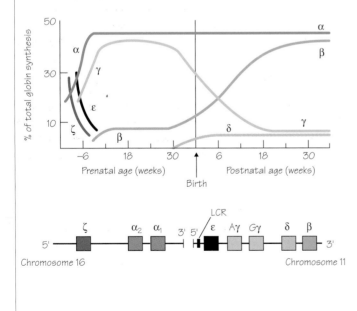

(c) The p50 is the partial pressure of oxygen at which haemoglobin is 50% saturated (red curve, normally 27mmHg). Decreased oxygen affinity, with increasing p50 (green curve) occurs as carbon dioxide concentration increases or pH decreases (Bohr effect) or 2,3-DPG levels rise. Increased oxygen affinity occurs during the opposite circumstances or may be a characteristic of a variant haemoglobin, which may lead to polycythaemia (see Chapter 27), e.g. Hb Chesapeake or Hb F.

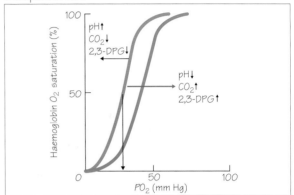

(d) Red cell metabolism.

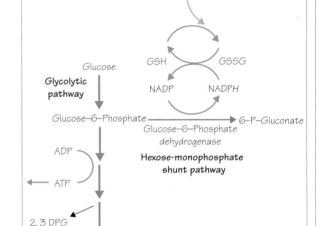

Peripheral blood cells

Normal peripheral blood contains mainly mature cells which do not undergo further division.

Red cells (erythrocytes)

Red cells are the most numerous of the peripheral blood cells (10^{12}/L). They are among the simplest of cells in vertebrates

Table 2.1 Normal haemoglobins

	Hb A	Hb A$_2$	Hb F
Structure	$\alpha_2\beta_2$	$\alpha_2\delta_2$	$\alpha_2\gamma_2$
Normal adult (%)	96–98	1.5–3.5	0.5–0.8

and are highly specialized for their function, which is to carry oxygen to all parts of the body and return carbon dioxide to the lungs. Red cells exist only within the circulation – unlike many types of white blood cells, they cannot traverse the endothelial membrane. They are larger than the diameter of the capillaries in the microcirculation. This requires them to have a flexible membrane. Red cells contain haemoglobin which allows them to carry oxygen (O_2) and carbon dioxide (CO_2). Haemoglobin is composed of four polypeptide globin chains each with an iron containing haem molecule (Fig. 2a). Embryonic haemoglobins (Portland, Gower I and II) are present in early foetal life, whereas foetal haemoglobin (Hb F, $\alpha_2\gamma_2$) dominates by late foetal life. Hb F has a higher oxygen affinity than Hb A, and this allows the foetus to obtain oxygen from the mother. A switch occurs at 3–6 months in the neonatal period to normal adult haemoglobin (Hb A) (Fig. 2b). Low levels of Hb F and the minor adult haemoglobin Hb A$_2$ ($\alpha_2\delta_2$) are present in normal adults (Table 2.1).

The ability of haemoglobin to bind O_2 is measured as the haemoglobin–O_2 dissociation curve. Raised concentrations of 2,3-DPG, H^+ ions or CO_2 decrease O_2 affinity, allowing more O_2 delivery to tissues (Fig. 2c). Some pathological variant haemoglobins are similar to Hb F in having a higher oxygen affinity than Hb A; this leads, in adults, to a state of relative tissue hypoxia and the body compensates by increasing the number of red cells (secondary polycythaemia, see Chapter 27). In contrast, some pathological variant haemoglobins (e.g. Hb S, the major haemoglobin in sickle cell disease, see Chapter 19) have a lower oxygen affinity than Hb A, and this allows individuals to maintain a higher level of tissue oxygenation for a given level of haemoglobin concentration.

Erythropoietin controls the production of red cells. It is produced in the peritubular complex of the kidney (90%), liver and other organs. Erythropoietin stimulates mixed lineage and red cell progenitors as well as pronormoblasts and early erythroblasts to proliferate, differentiate and produce haemoglobin (Table 2.1). Erythropoietin secretion is stimulated by reduced O_2 supply to the kidney receptor (see Table 27.1). Thus, the principal stimuli to red cell production are tissue hypoxia and reduced haemoglobin concentration (anaemia). Exogenous erythropoietin binds to the erythropoietin receptor on the surface of the red cell and induces signal transduction (see Fig. 1b) via phosphorylation of the Janus kinase 2 (JAK 2). This in turn induces gene transcription and red cell proliferation. Mutations in JAK 2 are known to underlie pathologically increased red cell production in polycythaemia rubra vera (PRV, see Chapter 26).

Developing red cells in the marrow (erythroblasts) are nucleated (see Fig. 8c); the nucleus condenses with maturation, to be extruded prior to red cell release into the circulation. **Reticulocytes** (Fig. 10b) are young non-nucleated red cells which retain RNA (stainable by supravital stains, i.e. stains used while the cells are still alive). They increase in number following acute haemorrhage, treatment of haematinic deficiency and in haemolytic anaemias. They are a measure of red cell production and of the age of the red cell population. Ten to fifteen per cent of developing erythroblasts die within the marrow without producing mature red cells. Increased '**ineffective erythropoiesis**' is an important cause of reduced haemoglobin concentration (anaemia) in various pathological states, e.g. thalassaemia major, myelofibrosis and megaloblastic anaemia.

Red cell metabolism

Red cells are capable of only the simplest metabolic pathways.

The glycolytic pathway (Fig. 2d) is the main source of energy (ATP) required to maintain red cell shape and deformability. The *hexose monophosphate* 'shunt' pathway provides the main source of reduced nicotinamide adenine dinucleotide phosphate (NADPH), which maintains reduced glutathione (GSH) and protects haemoglobin and the membrane proteins against oxidant damage. Oxygen radicals are freely generated by the constant oxygenation and deoxygenation of haemoglobin. Mature red cells have no nucleus, ribosomes or mitochondria. They survive for about 120 days before being removed by macrophages of the reticuloendothelial system (see Chapter 4).

The red cell membrane is a bipolar lipid layer which anchors surface antigens. It has a protein skeleton (spectrin, actin, protein 4.1 and ankyrin) which maintains the red cell's biconcave shape and deformability. These proteins contain several sulphydryl (-SH) groups which are essential for the maintenance of their tertiary structure and, therefore, the structural integrity of the red cell. These sulphydryl groups require NADPH generated by the pentose phosphate pathway to protect them from oxygen radicals.

Haematinics

Haematinics are naturally occurring substances, absorbed from the diet, which are essential for red cell production. They include minerals (e.g. iron) and vitamins (e.g. B$_{12}$, B$_6$ and folic acid).

Normal blood cells II: granulocytes, monocytes and the reticuloendothelial system

3

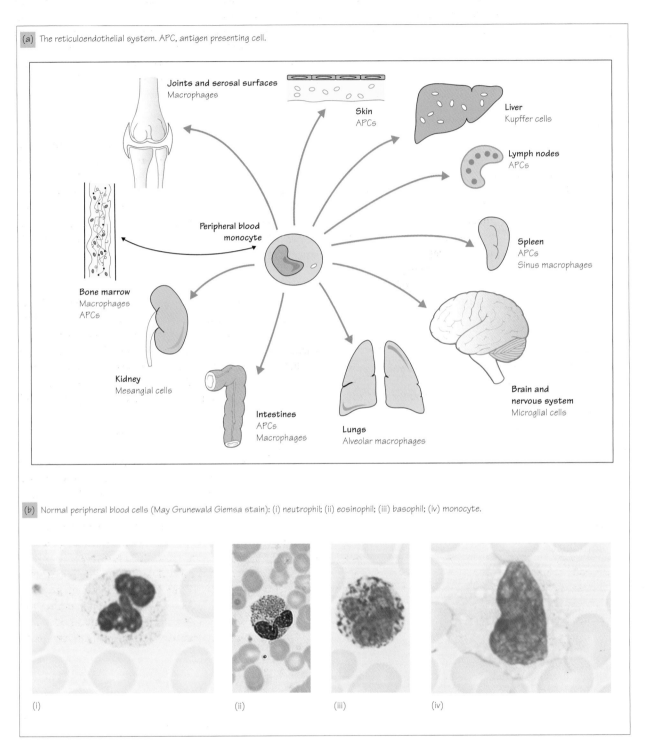

(a) The reticuloendothelial system. APC, antigen presenting cell.

Joints and serosal surfaces
Macrophages

Skin
APCs

Liver
Kupffer cells

Lymph nodes
APCs

Peripheral blood
monocyte

Spleen
APCs
Sinus macrophages

Bone marrow
Macrophages
APCs

Kidney
Mesangial cells

Intestines
APCs
Macrophages

Lungs
Alveolar macrophages

Brain and
nervous system
Microglial cells

(b) Normal peripheral blood cells (May Grunewald Giemsa stain): (i) neutrophil; (ii) eosinophil; (iii) basophil; (iv) monocyte.

(i)   (ii)   (iii)   (iv)

Normal white blood cells (leucocytes) in peripheral blood are of five types: three of them contain granules and termed granulocytes (neutrophils or polymorphonuclear granulocytes, eosinophils and basophils). The other two types are monocytes and lymphocytes (see Chapter 4). Granulocyte and monocyte production occurs in the bone marrow and is controlled by growth factors (see Table 1.1). External stimuli (e.g. infection, fever, inflammation, allergy, and trauma) act on cytokine networks to increase the production of these growth factors, e.g. IL-1 and TNF. The earliest recognizable granulocyte precursors are myeloblasts. These undergo a final division followed by further maturation into promyelocytes, myelocytes, metamyelocytes and, finally, mature granulocytes (neutrophils, eosinophils and basophils). Primary granules, present in promyelocytes, contain lysosomal enzymes. Secondary granules containing other enzymes (peroxidase, lysosyme, alkaline phosphatase and lactoferrin) appear later. Basophil granules contain histamine and heparin.

Function of white cells

The primary function of white cells is to protect the body against infection. They work closely with proteins of the immune response, immunoglobulins and complement. Neutrophils, eosinophils, basophils and monocytes are all phagocytes; they ingest and destroy pathogens and cell debris. Phagocytes are attracted to bacteria at the site of inflammation by chemotactic substances released from damaged tissues and by complement components. Opsonization is the coating of cells or foreign particles by immunoglobulin or complement; this aids phagocytosis (engulfment) because phagocytes have immunoglobulin Fc and complement C3b receptors (see below). Killing involves reduction of pH within the phagocytic vacuole, the release of granule contents and the production of antimicrobial oxidants and superoxides (the 'respiratory burst').

Neutrophils

Neutrophils (polymorphs) (Fig. 3b(i)) are the most numerous peripheral blood leucocytes. They have a short lifespan of around 10 hours in the circulation. About 50% of neutrophils in peripheral blood are attached to the walls of blood vessels (marginating pool). Neutrophils enter tissues by migrating in response to chemotactic factors. Migration, phagocytosis and killing are energy-dependent functions. The concentration of neutrophils in the blood may be lower in certain racial populations, e.g. black, Middle Eastern.

Eosinophils

Eosinophils have similar kinetics of production, differentiation and circulation to neutrophils; the growth factor IL-5 is important in regulating their production. They have a bilobed nucleus (Fig. 3b(ii)) and red-orange staining granules (containing histamine). They are particularly important in the response to parasitic and allergic diseases. Release of their granule contents onto larger pathogens (e.g. helminths) aids their destruction and subsequent phagocytosis.

Basophils

Basophils are closely related to mast cells (small darkly staining cells in the bone marrow and tissues). Both are derived from granulocyte precursors in the bone marrow. They are the least numerous of peripheral blood leucocytes and have large dark purple granules which may obscure the nucleus (Fig. 3b(iii)). The granule contents include histamine and heparin and are released following binding of IgE to surface receptors. They play an important part in immediate hypersensitivity reactions. Mast cells also have an important role in defence against allergens and parasitic pathogens.

Monocytes

Monocytes (Fig. 3b(iv)) circulate for 20–40 hours and then enter tissues as macrophages where they mature and carry out their principal functions. Within tissues, they survive for many days, possibly months. They have variable morphology in peripheral blood, but are mononuclear, have greyish cytoplasm with vacuoles and small granules. Within tissues, they often have long cytoplasmic projections allowing them to communicate widely with other cells.

Reticuloendothelial system

This is used to describe monocyte-derived cells (Fig. 3a) which are distributed throughout the body in multiple organs and tissues. The system includes Kupffer's cells in the liver, alveolar macrophages in the lung, mesangial cells in the kidney, microglial cells in the brain and macrophages within the bone marrow, spleen, lymph nodes, skin and serosal surfaces. The principal functions of the reticuloendothelial system (RES) are to

- phagocytose and destroy pathogens and cellular debris, e.g. red cell debris;
- process and present antigens to lymphoid cells (the antigen presenting cells react principally with T cells with whom they 'interdigitate' in lymph nodes, spleen, thymus, bone marrow and tissues);
- produce cytokines (e.g. IL-1) which regulate and participate within cytokine and growth factor networks governing haemopoiesis, inflammation and cellular responses.

The cells of the RES are particularly localized in tissues which may come into contact with external allergens or pathogens. The main organs of the RES allow its cells to communicate with lymphoid cells, and include the liver, spleen, lymph nodes, bone marrow, thymus and intestinal tract-associated lymphoid tissue.

4 Normal blood cells III: lymphocytes

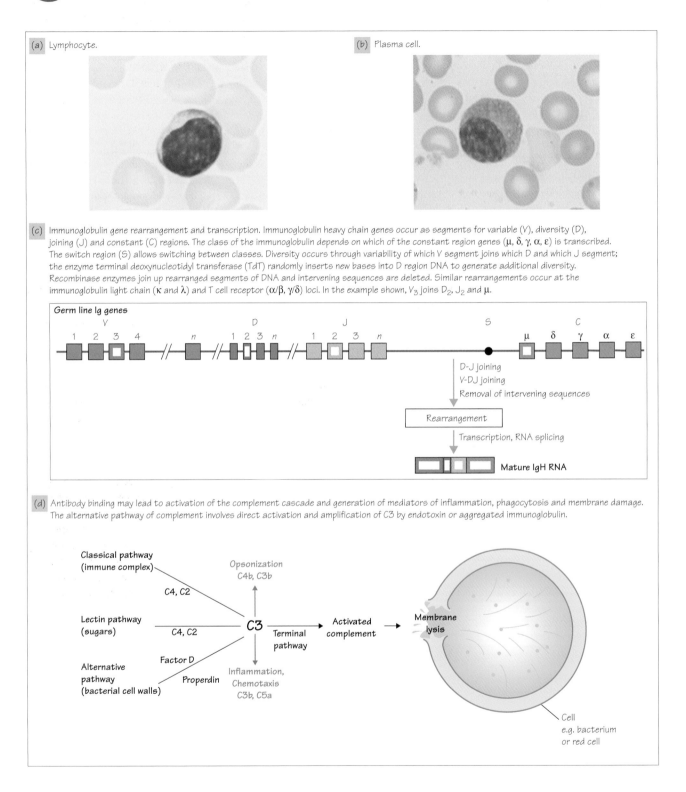

(a) Lymphocyte.

(b) Plasma cell.

(c) Immunoglobulin gene rearrangement and transcription. Immunoglobulin heavy chain genes occur as segments for variable (V), diversity (D), joining (J) and constant (C) regions. The class of the immunoglobulin depends on which of the constant region genes (μ, δ, γ, α, ϵ) is transcribed. The switch region (S) allows switching between classes. Diversity occurs through variability of which V segment joins which D and which J segment; the enzyme terminal deoxynucleotidyl transferase (TdT) randomly inserts new bases into D region DNA to generate additional diversity. Recombinase enzymes join up rearranged segments of DNA and intervening sequences are deleted. Similar rearrangements occur at the immunoglobulin light chain (κ and λ) and T cell receptor (α/β, γ/δ) loci. In the example shown, V_3 joins D_2, J_2 and μ.

(d) Antibody binding may lead to activation of the complement cascade and generation of mediators of inflammation, phagocytosis and membrane damage. The alternative pathway of complement involves direct activation and amplification of C3 by endotoxin or aggregated immunoglobulin.

Lymphocytes are an essential component of the immune response and are derived from haemopoietic stem cells. A common lymphoid stem cell undergoes differentiation and proliferation to give rise to B cells, which mediate humoral or antibody-mediated immunity, and T cells (processed in the thymus), responsible for cell-mediated immunity. Mature lymphocytes are small mononuclear cells with scanty blue cytoplasm (Fig. 4a). The majority of peripheral blood lymphocytes (70%) are T cells, which may have more cytoplasm than B cells and may contain granules.

Lymphocyte maturation occurs principally in bone marrow for B cells and in the thymus for T cells, but also involves the lymph nodes, liver, spleen and other parts of the reticuloendothelial system. Lymphocytes can be characterized on the basis of the antigens expressed on the surface of the cell. These differ according to the lineage and level of maturity of the cell. The cluster of differentiation (CD) nomenclature system has evolved as a means of classifying these antigens according to their reaction with monoclonal antibodies (see Appendix II). Lymphocytes have the longest lifespan of any leucocyte, and some (e.g. 'memory' B cells) live for many years.

Immune response

The immune response involves a complex interaction of cells (including B lymphocytes, T lymphocytes, macrophages), proteins (immunoglobulins, complement) and lipids (e.g. glycosphingolipids) whereby the body responds to infection, injury and neoplasia. Inflammation is a non-specific outcome of the immune response. Specificity of the immune response derives from amplification of antigen-selected T and B cells. The mature B cells that manufacture immunoglobulin are termed plasma cells (Fig. 4b). The T cell receptor (TCR) on T cells and surface membrane immunoglobulin (sIg) on B cells are receptor molecules which have a variable and a constant portions. The variability ensures that a specific antigen is recognized by a lymphocyte with a matching variable receptor region. The genetic mechanisms required to generate the required diversity are common to T and B cells (Fig. 4c). They involve rearrangement of variable, joining, diversity and constant region genes to generate genes coding for surface receptors (Ig or TCR) capable of reacting specifically with one of an enormous array of antigens.

The generation of a specific immune response involves interaction between antigens and T cells, B cells and antigen presenting cells (APCs), which are specialized macrophages. Mature T cells are of three main types: helper cells express the CD4 antigen and generally augment B cell responses; suppressor cells express CD8 and generally suppress B cells; and cytotoxic cells also expressing CD8. Developing T cells are 'educated' in the thymus only to react to foreign antigens, and to develop tolerance to self-human leucocyte antigens (HLA). B cells can also interact directly with antigen. Adhesion molecules mediate these cellular interactions. Reaction between antigen and appropriate receptor (sIg or TCR) leads to B or T cellular proliferation (clonal selection) and differentiation. A key location for clonal selection is the germinal centre of lymph nodes and spleen. 'Pre-germinal centre' B cells are less mature and have not undergone further mutation of nucleotide residues at the heavy chain variable region (VH) gene locus. More mature B cells are 'post-germinal centre' and have mutated VH genes. B cell malignancies derived from these B cells (e.g. chronic lymphocytic leukaemia, CLL, see Chapter 29) will reproduce this feature, and it is noteworthy that the degree of somatic mutation at the IgH immunoglobulin gene locus relates to prognosis of the leukaemia. Malignancies derived from very immature lymphocytes (e.g. B and T cell-derived acute lymphoblastic leukaemia, ALL, see Chapter 22) are generally positive for the enzyme TdT (terminal deoxynucleotidyl transferase) which is responsible for the generation of genetic diversity in B or T cells.

Natural killer cells

Natural killer cells are neither T nor B cells, though are often CD8$^+$. They characteristically have prominent granules and are often large granular lymphocytes. These cells are not governed by HLA restriction and can kill target cells by direct adhesion.

Immunoglobulins

These are gammaglobulins produced by plasma cells. There are five main groups: IgG, IgM, IgA, IgD and IgE. Each is composed of light and heavy chains, and each chain is made up of variable, joining and constant regions (Fig. 4c).

Complement

This is a group of plasma proteins and cell surface receptors which, if activated, interact with cellular and humoral elements in the inflammatory response (Fig. 4d). The complete molecule is capable of direct lysis of cell membranes and of pathogens sensitized by antibody. The C3b component coats cells making them sensitive to phagocytosis by macrophages. C3a and C5a may also activate chemotaxis by phagocytes and activate mast cells and basophils to release mediators of inflammation.

Lymph nodes, the lymphatic system and the spleen

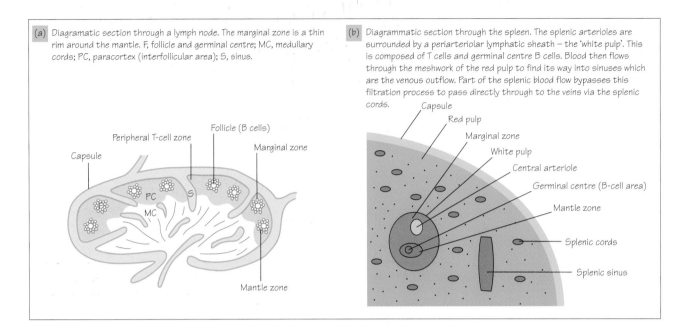

(a) Diagramatic section through a lymph node. The marginal zone is a thin rim around the mantle. F, follicle and germinal centre; MC, medullary cords; PC, paracortex (interfollicular area); S, sinus.

(b) Diagrammatic section through the spleen. The splenic arterioles are surrounded by a periarteriolar lymphatic sheath – the 'white pulp'. This is composed of T cells and germinal centre B cells. Blood then flows through the meshwork of the red pulp to find its way into sinuses which are the venous outflow. Part of the splenic blood flow bypasses this filtration process to pass directly through to the veins via the splenic cords.

The lymph nodes and spleen are important organs of the body's immune system and reticuloendothelial system (RES). They are key areas where antigen (processed by the cells of the RES) can be presented in proximity to the cells of the immune system (B cells and T cells). The anatomy of lymph nodes and spleen are illustrated in Figs. 5a and 5b. A common feature is the presence of germinal centres, which are an important location for B cell maturation and proliferation. The spleen has a specialized circulatory network which allows it to perform its functions. Red cells are concentrated from the arteriolar circulation and pass through the endothelial meshwork of the red pulp to the sinuses of the venous circulation. This process brings antigens, particulate matter (e.g. opsonized bacteria), effete cells or unwanted material from within deformable red cells (e.g. nuclear remnants, iron granules) in proximity with the specialized cells of the RES, the splenic macrophages. These macrophages and lymphocytes occupy the densely cellular areas of the spleen termed the white pulp.

Lymph and the lymphatic system

Lymph is a fluid which is derived from blood as a filtrate and circulates around the body (including lymph nodes, liver, spleen and serosal surfaces) in lymph vessels (the lymphatic system). Lymph is rich in lymphocytes, which are returned to the blood circulation via the azygous vein and thoracic duct which return lymph to the right atrium. Obstruction of the lymph vessels (e.g. by external compression or as a result of pathology within lymph nodes) leads to swelling (oedema or lymphoedema). Causes of lymph node enlargement are listed in Table 5.1.

Functions of the spleen

The spleen is a specialized organ with an anatomical structure designed to allow antigens which are circulating in the systemic blood stream or have been absorbed from the gastrointestinal tract into the portal circulation to be processed by macrophages of the RES and presented to the cells of the immune system. The functions of the spleen are
- to allow antigens to be processed and presented to lymphoid cells;
- to manufacture antibody;
- to allow antibody-coated cells to be phagocytosed by the interaction with macrophages via their surface Fe receptors;

Table 5.1 Causes of lymphadenopathy

Local
Localized bacterial/viral infection
Skin condition, e.g. trauma, eczema
Malignant – secondary carcinoma, lymphoma

General
Infection
bacterial, e.g. endocarditis, tuberculosis
viral, e.g. HIV, infectious mononucleosis, cytomegalovirus
other, e.g. toxoplasmosis, malaria
Malignancy
e.g. lymphoma, lymphoid leukaemias
Inflammatory disorders
e.g. sarcoidosis, connective tissue diseases
Generalized allergic conditions
e.g. widespread eczema

- to temporarily sequester red cells (especially reticulocytes) and allow removal of nuclear remnants, siderotic (iron-containing) granules and other inclusions;
- haemopoiesis in early foetal life; and (rarely) in some pathological rates, e.g. myelofibrosis.

Impaired splenic function or splenectomy reduces the body's ability to make antibody (particularly to capsulated organisms, e.g. pneumococcus, haemophilus, meningococcus), reduces clearance of intracellular organisms (e.g. parasitized red cells) and impairs defence against organisms and toxins in the portal circulation. Splenic function may be impaired due to congenital absence of the spleen. Acquired hyposplenism occurs when there is recurrent thrombosis affecting the arterial systemic blood flow to the spleen (e.g. sickle cell disease, essential thrombocythaemia), infiltration of the spleen (e.g. amyloid), in gluten-induced enteropathy and less frequently inflammatory bowel disease or in the presence of high levels of circulating immune complexes (e.g. autoimmune diseases).

Splenomegaly

Causes of an enlarged spleen are listed in Table 5.2. Inflammation and infection typically cause an increase in the white cell areas (white pulp), while congestion causes an increase in the red cell areas (red pulp). Proliferation of malignant cells, infiltration, storage disease and extramedullary haemopoiesis are other causes of enlargement.

Splenectomy

Splenectomy is beneficial in a number of haematological conditions, particularly when the spleen is the site of excessive destruction of peripheral blood cells, e.g. selected patients with haemolytic anaemia and thrombocytopenia (particularly autoimmune), and myelofibrosis. The spleen has an important role

Table 5.2 Causes of splenomegaly

Haemolytic anaemia
Hereditary spherocytosis, autoimmune haemolytic anaemia, thalassaemia major or intermedia, sickle cell anaemia (before infarction occurs)

Haematological malignancies
Lymphoma, CLL, ALL, AML, CML*
Polycythaemia vera, myelofibrosis*
Myelodysplasia

Storage diseases
Gaucher's*
Amyloid

Liver disease and portal hypertension
Congestive cardiac failure
Infection
Malaria*
Leishmaniasis*
Bacterial endocarditis
Viral infections, e.g. infectious mononucleosis

ALL, acute lymphoblastic leukaemia; AML, acute myeloid leukaemia; CLL, chronic lymphocytic leukaemia; CML, chronic myeloid leukaemia
*Causes of massive splenomegaly

in removing capsulated and opsonized bacteria (see Chapter 3), and splenectomy (or hyposplenism due to disease, see above) leads to an increased susceptibility to infection. The operation should be avoided in children below 5 years and should be preceded by vaccination against pneumococcus, haemophilus influenza type B and meningococcus. Patients who are hyposplenic or post-splenectomy should take prophylactic antibiotics indefinitely (e.g. oral penicillin V or erythromycin at low dose) and should carry a card at all times informing of their condition. Malaria is also likely to be more severe.

6 Clinical assessment

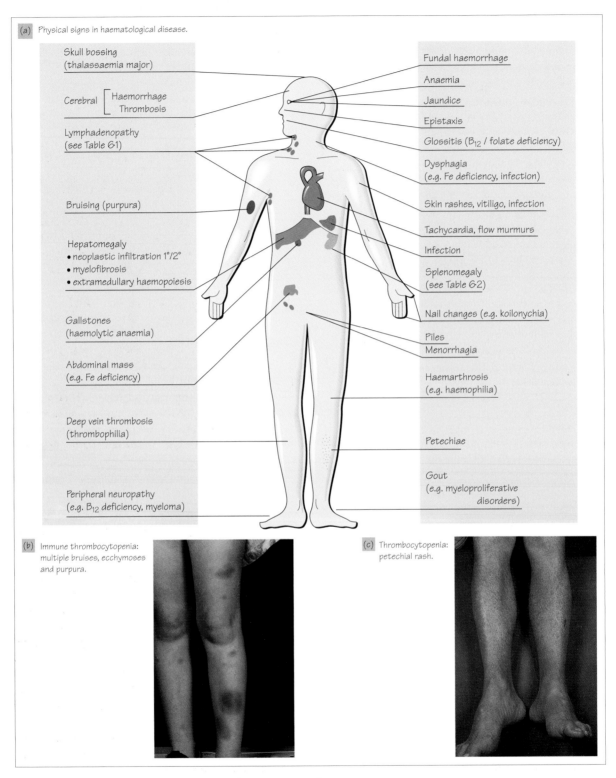

(a) Physical signs in haematological disease.

Skull bossing (thalassaemia major)

Cerebral ⎡ Haemorrhage
⎣ Thrombosis

Lymphadenopathy (see Table 6·1)

Bruising (purpura)

Hepatomegaly
• neoplastic infiltration 1°/2°
• myelofibrosis
• extramedullary haemopoiesis

Gallstones (haemolytic anaemia)

Abdominal mass (e.g. Fe deficiency)

Deep vein thrombosis (thrombophilia)

Peripheral neuropathy (e.g. B_{12} deficiency, myeloma)

Fundal haemorrhage

Anaemia

Jaundice

Epistaxis

Glossitis (B_{12} / folate deficiency)

Dysphagia (e.g. Fe deficiency, infection)

Skin rashes, vitiligo, infection

Tachycardia, flow murmurs

Infection

Splenomegaly (see Table 6·2)

Nail changes (e.g. koilonychia)

Piles
Menorrhagia

Haemarthrosis (e.g. haemophilia)

Petechiae

Gout (e.g. myeloproliferative disorders)

(b) Immune thrombocytopenia: multiple bruises, ecchymoses and purpura.

(c) Thrombocytopenia: petechial rash.

Haematological illness leads to a range of symptoms and signs which are described in this chapter. An accurate history, careful clinical examination and appropriate laboratory assessment are essential for successful management of patients.

History

Anaemia

This is a reduction in the concentration of haemoglobin which leads to reduced oxygen carriage and delivery.

18 *Haematology at a Glance*, 3e. By A. Mehta and V. Hoffbrand. Published 2009 by Blackwell Publishing. ISBN 978-1-4051-7970-6.

- Symptoms: shortness of breath on exertion, tiredness, headache or angina, more marked if anaemia is severe, of rapid onset and in older subjects.
- Causes: e.g. bleeding, dietary deficiency, malabsorption, systemic illness, haemolysis, bone marrow failure, inherited abnormalities of red cells.

Leucopenia

This is a reduction in white cell number which, if severe, predisposes to infection. It may be due to the following:
- Neutropenia, particularly if neutrophils are $<0.5 \times 10^9$/L, which frequently leads to bacterial or fungal infection in skin, mouth, throat and chest. Pus is lacking.
- Infection is often atypical, caused by organisms non-pathogenic for normal individuals, rapidly progressive and difficult to treat.
- Lymphopenia which reduces B and T cell (humoral and T cell-mediated) immunity and predisposes particularly to viral infection (e.g. herpes zoster), tuberculosis, protozoal and fungal infections.
- Functional defects of neutrophils and lymphocytes also predispose to infection.

Thrombocytopenia

This is a reduction in blood platelets which leads to an increased tendency to bruising and bleeding (Figs. 6b and 6c).
- Spontaneous bruises (purpura) which may be raised (ecchymoses) or small pin-sized capillary haemorrhages (petechiae), mucosal bleeding, e.g. epistaxis, menorrhagia. Bleeding following trauma is increased with platelets $<50 \times 10^9$/L. Spontaneous bleeding occurs when platelets $<10 \times 10^9$/L.
- Functional platelet defects also predispose to bleeding.

  NB: Combination of anaemia, excessive bleeding and/or infection suggest pancytopenia caused by bone marrow failure (see Chapter 18).

Coagulation factor defects

- Easy bleeding after trauma (e.g. circumcision, dental treatment), spontaneous haemorrhage in deep tissues (e.g. muscles, joints), family history.
- Acquired coagulation defects often accompanied by thrombocytopenia lead to spontaneous skin bleeding and excessive bleeding in response to trauma.

Other symptoms (Fig. 6a)

- Weight loss, fever, pruritus and skin rash – lymphoma or myeloproliferative disorder.
- Bone pain, symptoms of hypercalcaemia (thirst, polyuria, constipation) – myeloma.
- Left hypochondrial pain – splenomegaly.
- Painless lymphadenopathy suggests malignancy, whereas painful may indicate inflammation/infection.
- Joint pains – gout caused by hyperuricaemia.

Family history

Inherited anaemia (e.g. genetic disorders of haemoglobin), coagulation disorders (e.g. haemophilia) and certain leucocyte and platelet disorders.

Drug history

Haemolytic anaemia in G6PD deficiency, disordered platelet function caused by aspirin, drug-induced agranulocytosis, macrocytosis of red cells caused by alcohol.

Operations

Gastrectomy, intestinal resection may lead to iron or vitamin B_{12} deficiency. Splenectomy may lead to infection.

Examination

- Pallor of mucous membranes, if Hb < 9 g/dL, indicates anaemia.
- Tachycardia, systolic murmur (cardiac output and pulse rate rise to compensate for anaemia).
- Jaundice (haemolytic or megaloblastic anaemia), pigment gallstones.
- Lymphadenopathy (generalized or localized) (see Table 5.1).
- Skin changes, e.g. purpura caused by thrombocytopenia, vitiligo associated with pernicious anaemia, melanin pigmentation in iron overload, ankle ulcers in haemolytic anaemia, rashes caused by tumour infiltration.
- Nail changes (e.g. koilonychia in iron deficiency).
- Signs of infection (mouth, throat, skin, perineum, chest) associated with neutropenia.
- Mouth, e.g. angular cheilosis in iron deficiency, glossitis in B_{12} or folate deficiency.
- Hepatomegaly or splenomegaly (see Table 5.2).
- Nervous system examination, e.g. B_{12} neuropathy, peripheral neuropathy in myeloma, amyloidosis, malignant infiltration in central nervous system leukaemia or lymphoma.
- Optic fundi, e.g. haemorrhage in severe anaemia, hyperviscosity in polycythaemia.

Special investigations

Haematological diseases are often multisystem disorders and a range of special investigations (X-ray, ultrasound, CT/MRI imaging, endoscopy, etc.) is frequently required to define the extent and stage of the disease.

Nuclear medicine studies allow study of organ function, and tests useful to haematologists include the following.
- Isotope labelling of cells followed by scanning, e.g. autologous red cells can be labelled with radioactive chromium/technetium, reinjected and their lifespan measured, loss detected in stools and destruction in liver/spleen detected by surface counting. Labelled white cell (gallium) scans can detect occult infection or lymphoma. Labelled platelet scans can measure platelet lifespan and destruction in liver/spleen can be quantified.
- Positron emission tomography (PET) measures metabolic activity of tissue and is able to distinguish active tumour, e.g. lymphoma (positive) from inactive scar tissue (negative) after chemotherapy or radiotherapy.
- Multiple gated acquisition (MUGA) scanning to assess left ventricular function (impaired due to chemotherapy, radiotherapy or iron overload).

  Laboratory tests are described in Chapter 7.

7 Laboratory assessment

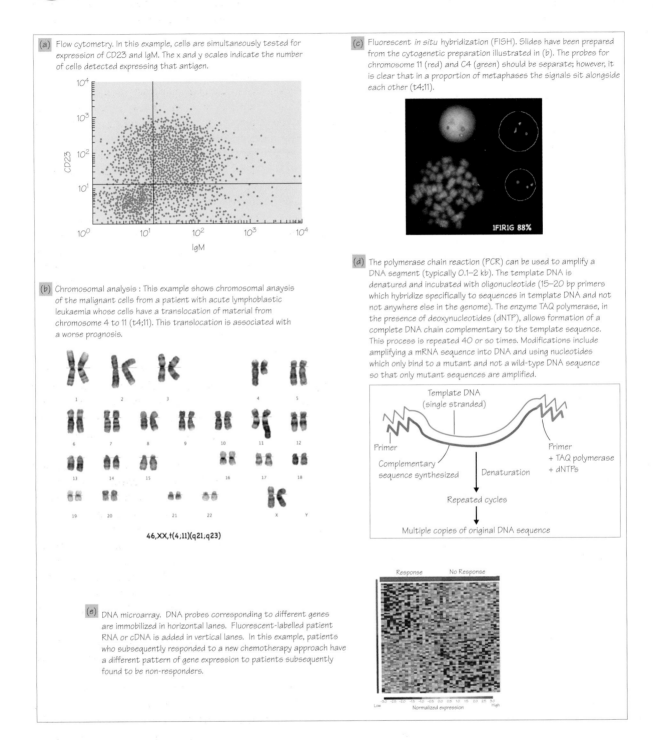

(a) Flow cytometry. In this example, cells are simultaneously tested for expression of CD23 and IgM. The x and y scales indicate the number of cells detected expressing that antigen.

(c) Fluorescent *in situ* hybridization (FISH). Slides have been prepared from the cytogenetic preparation illustrated in (b). The probes for chromosome 11 (red) and C4 (green) should be separate; however, it is clear that in a proportion of metaphases the signals sit alongside each other (t4;11).

1F1R1G 88%

(b) Chromosomal analysis : This example shows chromosomal anaysis of the malignant cells from a patient with acute lymphoblastic leukaemia whose cells have a translocation of material from chromosome 4 to 11 (t4;11). This translocation is associated with a worse prognosis.

46,XX,t(4;11)(q21;q23)

(d) The polymerase chain reaction (PCR) can be used to amplify a DNA segment (typically 0.1–2 kb). The template DNA is denatured and incubated with oligonucleotide (15–20 bp primers which hybridize specifically to sequences in template DNA and not not anywhere else in the genome). The enzyme TAQ polymerase, in the presence of deoxynucleotides (dNTP), allows formation of a complete DNA chain complementary to the template sequence. This process is repeated 40 or so times. Modifications include amplifying a mRNA sequence into DNA and using nucleotides which only bind to a mutant and not a wild-type DNA sequence so that only mutant sequences are amplified.

Template DNA (single stranded)

Primer
Complementary sequence synthesized
Denaturation
Primer + TAQ polymerase + dNTPs

Repeated cycles

Multiple copies of original DNA sequence

(e) DNA microarray. DNA probes corresponding to different genes are immobilized in horizontal lanes. Fluorescent-labelled patient RNA or cDNA is added in vertical lanes. In this example, patients who subsequently responded to a new chemotherapy approach have a different pattern of gene expression to patients subsequently found to be non-responders.

Response   No Response

Low   Normalized expression   High

Routine tests

Full blood count (see Appendix II)

Blood sample in sequestrene (ethylenediaminetetraacetate, EDTA) anticoagulant is tested by an automated analyzer (see Chapter 8). Analysers provide the following:

- Haemoglobin concentration, haematocrit, red cell count, red cell indices (see Chapter 10).

- White cell count and differential (neutrophils, lymphocytes, monocytes; eosinophils and basophils).
- Platelet count and size.
- Analysers also provide automated reticulocyte counts and enumerate immature platelets ('platelet reticulocytes').

Blood film

Blood film examination should be undertaken whenever the full blood count is abnormal, to assess red cell size/shape, white cell appearance and differential, abnormal cells, platelet size and morphology and detection of parasites, e.g. malaria.

Erythrocyte sedimentation rate, plasma/whole blood viscosity and C-reactive protein

The erythrocyte sedimentation rate (ESR) measures the rate of fall of a column of red cells in plasma in 1 hour. It is largely determined by plasma concentrations of proteins, especially fibrinogen and globulins. It is raised in anaemia. Normal range rises with age. A raised ESR is a non-specific indicator of an acute phase response and is of value in monitoring disease activity (e.g. rheumatoid arthritis). A raised ESR occurs in inflammatory disorders, infections, malignancy, myeloma, anaemia and pregnancy. The *plasma viscosity* gives comparable information but is less widely used. *Whole blood viscosity* is also influenced by the cell counts and is therefore raised when the red cell count (erythrocrit), white cell count (leucocrit) or platelet count is grossly raised. *C-reactive protein* is raised in an acute phase response and is valuable in monitoring this.

Bone marrow aspiration and trephine biopsy

See Chapter 8.

Specialized tests

These are discussed in the relevant chapter; some tests particularly used in the malignant haematological diseases are described here.

Flow cytometry

Flow cytometry (Fig. 7a) is an automated technique whereby a population of cells is incubated with specific monoclonal antibodies which are conjugated to a fluorochrome. The labelled cells are then passed in a fluid stream across a laser light source which allows quantitative analysis of antigen expression on the cell population. The technique is important in detecting and quantifying abnormal populations of cells, e.g. leukaemia diagnosis, assessment of residual malignant disease.

Chromosomal analysis

Normal individuals have 46 chromosomes: 44 autosomes (22 from each parent) and 2 sex chromosomes (46 XY = male, 46 XX = female). Chromosomal analysis is made initially by special stains of cells in division. Loss or gain of whole chromosomes, chromosome breaks and loss, inversion or translocation of a part of a chromosome can be detected (Fig. 7b). *Fluorescent in situ hybridization* (FISH) is a sensitive technique for detecting chromosome abnormalities (Fig. 7c) which involves the use of a fluorescent DNA probe which hybridizes selectively to a particular chromosome segment, allowing sensitive detection of deletion, translocation and duplication of that segment, or fusion with another chromosome. It has the advantage not only of detecting small abnormalities but being applicable to interphase (non-dividing cells).

DNA abnormalities

DNA abnormality as a cause of haematological disease may be inherited or acquired. *Inherited* haematological diseases are most commonly autosomal recessive, requiring an individual to inherit two mutant copies (alleles) of a gene (one from each parent) for expression of the disease (homozygotes). Carriers (heterozygotes) have one normal and one mutant allele and may express minor abnormalities clinically. Autosomal dominant diseases are rarer and require only one mutant allele for full expression of the disease. Sex-linked diseases arise if the mutant gene is on the X chromosome; males, having only one X chromosome, are affected, whereas females are carriers. *Acquired* DNA abnormalities are frequently present in clones of malignant cell populations and serve as disease markers and clues to pathogenesis (see Chapter 21).

Molecular techniques

These include the following:
- Southern blotting which allows assessment of deletion, rearrangement, inversion or duplication of DNA segments. Single base mutations will only be detected, however, if they alter the recognition sequence of a restriction enzyme. Southern blotting has now been largely replaced by polymerase chain reaction (PCR) techniques.
- PCR (Fig. 7d) can be used to amplify a DNA segment which can then be sequenced or digested by a restriction enzyme and fractionated by size using gel electrophoresis. PCR can be used to characterize a clone of malignant cells (minimal residual disease, see Chapter 21) or to diagnose inherited mutations (e.g. haemoglobin and coagulation disorders). It is used widely for antenatal diagnosis. PCR can be quantitative, e.g. 'real time' in which the number of cycles required to give a certain amount of DNA compared with a known standard is compared.
- Gene expression is studied by analysing RNA extracted from fresh cells, e.g. by gel electrophoresis (Northern blot). It can be semi-quantitated by using the enzyme reverse transcriptase to generate a DNA copy and then applying a modified PCR technique.
- DNA microarray analyses expression of multiple cellular genes (Fig. 7e). Fluorescent-labelled cell RNA or cDNA to be analysed is hybridized to DNA probes immobilized on a solid support. The pattern of mRNA expression is obtained, and this is characteristic of the different leukaemia or lymphoma subtype or prognostic group.

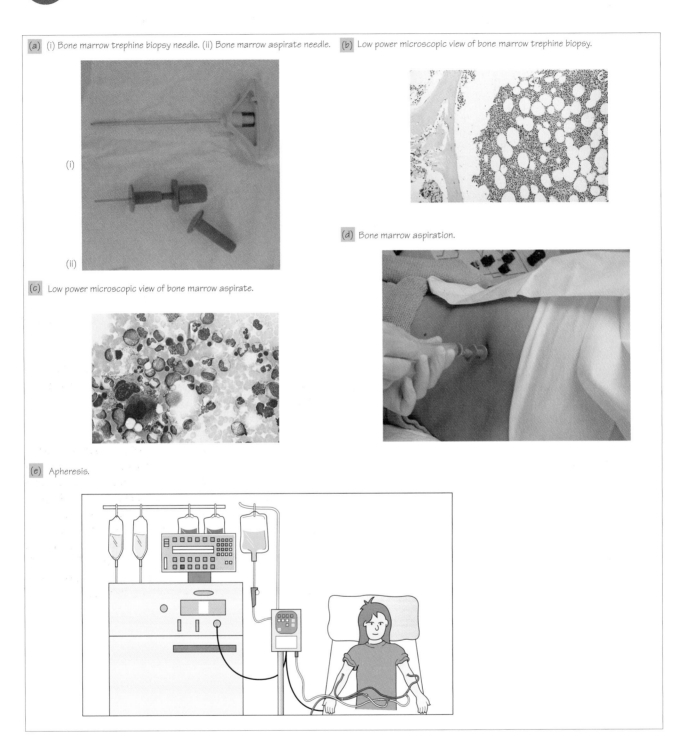

(a) (i) Bone marrow trephine biopsy needle. (ii) Bone marrow aspirate needle.

(b) Low power microscopic view of bone marrow trephine biopsy.

(i)

(ii)

(d) Bone marrow aspiration.

(c) Low power microscopic view of bone marrow aspirate.

(e) Apheresis.

Apheresis

Apheresis is a technique whereby whole blood is removed from the body and processed by centrifugation into its cellular components and plasma (Fig. 8e). In plasma exchange, the plasma is removed and replaced by albumin (or fresh frozen plasma in thrombotic thrombocytopenia purpura, TTP, see Chapter 37).

In *leucapheresis*, the white cells are removed. The process can also be used to perform a red cell exchange (e.g. in sickle cell disease), to remove platelets (platelet pheresis), to isolate lymphocytes for donation (donor lymphocyte infusion, DLI, e.g. for the treatment of relapse following a stem cell transplant) or to donate haemopoietic stem cells.

Table 8.1 Indications for bone marrow aspiration (and trephine)*

Unexplained cytopenia*
Anaemia, leucopenia, thrombocytopenia
Suspected marrow infiltrate*
Leukaemia, myelodysplasia, lymphoma, myeloproliferative disease, myeloma, carcinoma, storage disorders
Suspected infection
Leishmaniasis, tuberculosis

*Bone marrow trephine is required for pancytopenia or suspected marrow infiltration

Table 8.2 Special tests on bone marrow cells

Chromosomes
    Conventional cytogenetics, e.g. diagnosis and classification of leukaemia, myelodysplasia
FISH
    Detection of (submicroscopic) chromosome deletions, duplications, translocations, inversions
DNA analysis
    Detection and classification of
        leukaemia
        myeloproliferative diseases
        lymphoproliferative diseases
    Detection of residual disease
Immunophenotype analysis
    Diagnosis and classification of
        leukaemia
        lymphoproliferative diseases
        detection of residual disease
Gene assay analysis
    Diagnosis and classification of
        haematological malignant diseases
Microbiological cultures, e.g. tuberculosis
Cytochemistry – diagnosis of acute leukaemias

Bone marrow aspiration

Bone marrow is aspirated from the posterior iliac crest; a trephine biopsy is usually taken at the same time. Alternative sites for **aspiration** of marrow are the sternum and the medial part of the tibia (infants). The procedure is under local anaesthesia with or without intravenous sedation (Fig. 8d). Indications for marrow aspiration are listed in Table 8.1. Aspirated cells and particles of marrow are spread on slides (Fig. 8c), stained by Romanowsky stain and for iron (Perls' stain; see Fig. 12b). Specialized tests may also be performed (Table 8.2).

Bone marrow trephine biopsy

This is a more invasive procedure, using a larger needle (Fig. 8a) whereby a core of bone is biopsied from the iliac crest. This is then fixed in formalin and sections are cut. It is stained routinely by haematoxylin and eosin and a silver stain. Immunostaining is also performed if a haematological malignancy is suspected.

Lumbar Puncture

Cerebrospinal fluid is sampled from patients with haematological diseases for:

• Diagnosis – e.g. in case of infection; or infiltration by malignant cells.

• Treatment – e.g. malignancy (acute leukaemia, lymphoma) with intrathecal chemotherapy.

Lumbar puncture should be undertaken only in patients who have a platelet count $>50 \times 10^9$/L and after correction of coagulation abnormalities. Intrathecal chemotherapy should be prescribed and administered only by those who have appropriate training and experience.

Hickman line care

In-dwelling lines which have been tunnelled under the skin and then into the subclavian vein (see Chapter 49) allow easy venous access for blood sampling, administration of intravenous drugs, e.g. chemotherapy, antibiotics and feeding. All the ports must be kept patent by instillation of heparin when not in use. They should be sampled by wearing gloves and using sterile technique. The first 5–10 mL of blood from each port must be discarded before samples are sent for testing. If the tube is blocked, the installation of urokinase or alteplase (tissue plasminogen activator) is used to dissolve the thrombus.

Benign disorders of white cells: granulocytes, monocytes, macrophages and lymphocytes

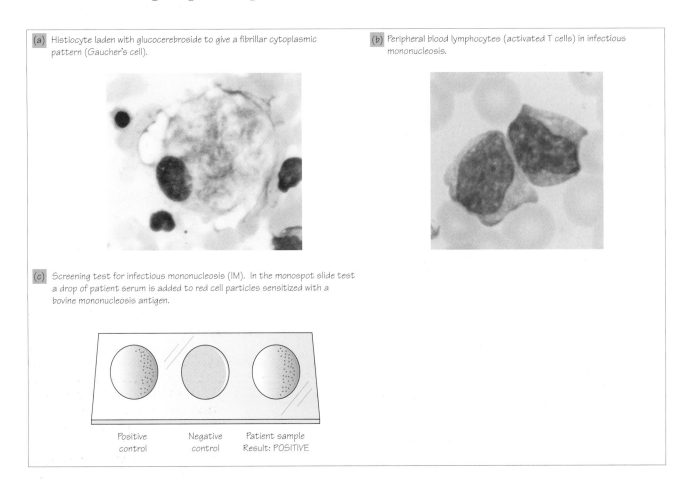

(a) Histiocyte laden with glucocerebroside to give a fibrillar cytoplasmic pattern (Gaucher's cell).

(b) Peripheral blood lymphocytes (activated T cells) in infectious mononucleosis.

(c) Screening test for infectious mononucleosis (IM). In the monospot slide test a drop of patient serum is added to red cell particles sensitized with a bovine mononucleosis antigen.

Positive control

Negative control

Patient sample
Result: POSITIVE

Granulocytes and monocytes

Inflammation commonly causes a **neutrophil leucocytosis (neutrophilia)** (Table 9.1). In addition, neutrophil granules may stain intensely (toxic granulation) and Doehle bodies (cytoplasmic RNA) may be present. A leukaemoid reaction is a profound reactive neutrophilia in which granulocyte precursors (e.g. myelocytes) appear in the blood. Neutropenia (reduced number of circulating neutrophils, see Table 9.2) increases susceptibility to infection, particularly bacterial. The normal neutrophil count is lower in black and Middle Eastern subjects than white people; this has no clinical consequences. Causes of **eosinophilia** are listed in Table 9.3. **Basophilia** (increase in blood basophils to >0.1 × 10⁹/L) is uncommon but occurs in myeloproliferative disorders. **Monocytosis** (increase in circulating monocytes to >1.0 × 10⁹/L) may occur in chronic infections (bacterial and protozoal, particularly in patients who cannot mount a neutrophil response), in malignancy and in myelodysplasia (see Chapter 25). **Disorders of neutrophil function** may be congenital or acquired and affect neutrophil interaction with immunoglobulin/complement, migration, phagocytosis and microbicidal activity. *Chronic granulomatous disease* is a rare inherited (X-linked) condition in which neutrophils are able to phagocytose but not kill. Acquired defects occur, for example, in diabetes, myelodysplasia and corticosteroid therapy.

Lysosomal storage disease

Hereditary deficiencies of enzymes required for glycolipid metabolism lead to the accumulation of ceramide components in various cells and tissues. *Gaucher's disease* is the most common (autosomal recessive) and is caused by mutations in the gene encoding glucocerebrosidase. Type I (most common) occurs especially among Ashkenazic Jews (age of presentation from infancy to middle age) and does not involve the central nervous system (CNS); types II and III are rarer and do involve the CNS. Clinical features (enlarged liver and spleen, characteristic bone defects) and haematological features (anaemia, thrombocytopenia with easy bruising) result from accumulation of Gaucher's cells (Fig. 9a) in the spleen, liver, skeleton, marrow and in types II and III in the CNS. Treatment is principally by enzyme replacement therapy.

24 *Haematology at a Glance*, 3e. By A. Mehta and V. Hoffbrand. Published 2009 by Blackwell Publishing. ISBN 978-1-4051-7970-6.

Table 9.1 Causes of neutrophilia (neutrophils >7.5 × 10⁹/L)

Bacterial infections
Inflammation, e.g. collagen diseases, Crohn's disease
Trauma/surgery
Tissue necrosis/infarction
Neoplasia
Haemorrhage and haemolysis
Metabolic, e.g. diabetic ketoacidosis
Myeloproliferative disorders
Myeloid leukaemias
Pregnancy
Drugs, e.g. steroids, GCSF

GCSF, granulocyte colony-stimulating factor

Table 9.2 Causes of neutropenia (neutrophils <1.5 × 10⁹/L)

1 Decreased production
  (a) General bone marrow failure, e.g. aplastic anaemia, megaloblastic anaemia, myelodysplasia, acute leukaemia, chemotherapy, replacement by tumour (see Chapter 18)
  (b) Specific failure of neutrophil production
     Congenital, e.g. Kostmann's syndrome
     Cyclical
     Drug-induced, e.g. sulphonamides, chlorpromazine, clozaril, diuretics, deferiprone, neomercazole, gold
     Viral infections
2 Increased destruction
  (a) General, e.g. hypersplenism
  (b) Specific, e.g. autoimmune – alone or in association with connective tissue disorder, rheumatoid arthritis (Felty's syndrome)

Normal black and Middle Eastern subjects have lower counts

Table 9.3 Causes of eosinophilia (eosinophils <1.5 × 10⁹/L)

Allergic diseases, e.g. asthma, hay fever, eczema, pulmonary hypersensitivity reaction (e.g. Loeffler's syndrome)

Parasitic disease

Skin diseases, e.g. psoriasis, drug rash

Drug sensitivity

Connective tissue disease

Haematological malignancy (e.g. Hodgkin lymphoma)

Idiopathic hypereosinophilia

Eosinophilic leukaemia (rare)

Histiocyte disorders

Histiocytes are the terminally differentiated cells of the monocyte/macrophage system and are widely distributed throughout all tissues. Langerhans cells are macrophages present in epidermis, spleen, thymus, bone, lymph nodes and mucosal surfaces. *Langerhans cell histiocytosis* (LCH) is a rare single organ or system or multisystem disease occurring princi-pally in childhood (<10 yr), with an incidence of two to three cases per million population. Clinical features include skin rash, bone pain/swelling, lymphadenopathy, hepatosplenomegaly, endocrine changes (e.g. diabetes insipidus as a result of posterior pituitary involvement) and skeletal lesions. Malignant histiocyte disorders include monocytic variants of acute leukaemia (see Chapter 22) and some types of non-Hodgkin lymphoma (see Chapter 32).

Haemophagocytic syndromes

In these syndromes, the bone marrow shows increased numbers of histiocytes which contain ingested blood cells, leading to pancytopenia. The mechanism is poorly understood and prognosis is usually poor. Causes include infection (viral, bacterial, tuberculosis), especially in an immunosuppressed host, tumours (e.g. lymphoma) (see Fig. 44a) or rare familial types.

Lymphocyte disorders

Lymphocytosis occurs in viral infections, some bacterial infections (e.g. pertussis) and in lymphoid neoplasia.

Lymphopenia (reduction in circulating lymphocytes to <1.5 × 10⁹/L) occurs in viral infection (e.g. HIV), lymphoma, connective tissue disease, severe bone marrow failure and with immunosuppressive drug therapy.

Infectious mononucleosis (*glandular fever*) is caused by Epstein–Barr virus (EBV) infection of B lymphocytes. Atypical circulating lymphocytes are reactive T cells. Cytomegalovirus, other viruses and toxoplasma infections cause a similar blood picture (Fig. 9b). Clinical features include onset usually in young adults (age 15–40 yr), sore throat, lymphadenopathy, fever, morbilliform rash – particularly following treatment with amoxicillin – and jaundice, hepatomegaly and tender splenomegaly in a minority. Complications include autoimmune thrombocytopenia and/or haemolytic anaemia, myocarditis, neuropathy, encephalitis, hepatitis and postviral fatigue syndrome. The Paul–Bunnell test, modified as the monospot slide test (Fig. 9c), detects heterophile antibodies (antibodies against cells of a different species). These agglutinate sheep red blood cells and, unlike those present in normal people, are not absorbed by guinea pig kidney cells, but are absorbed by ox red blood cells. The test is positive from 1 week after infection and persists for up to 2 months. Viral culture from sputum/saliva and specific IgM and IgG antibody tests against EBV nuclear and capsular antigens are sometimes useful in diagnosis.

Immunodeficiency

Depressed humoral immunity may be congenital (e.g. X-linked agammaglobulinaemia) or acquired (e.g. myeloma and chronic lymphocytic leukaemia, CLL) and characteristically leads to recurrent pyogenic bacterial infections. Depressed cell-mediated immunity may be congenital (e.g. DiGeorge's syndrome) or acquired (e.g. HIV infection, lymphoma, CLL) and causes susceptibility to viral, protozoal and fungal infections, anergy and a secondary defect in humoral immunity. Mixed B- and T-cell deficiency is common.

General aspects of red cells

(a) Automatic cell counter.

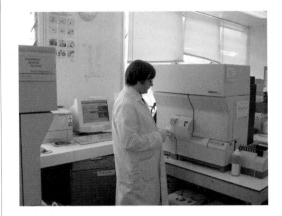

(b) Reticulocyte (brilliant cresyl blue stain) with blue strands of RNA.

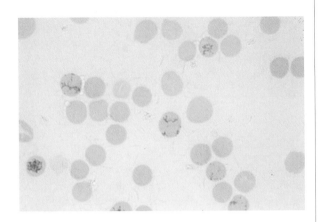

(c) Red cell morphology.

(d) High performance liquid chromatography. (i) HPLC printout showing a patient with β-thalassaemia trait – major band of HbA with increased concentrations of HbA2 and HbF. (ii) A patient with sickle cell trait and two bands corresponding to HbA and HbS.

Red cell abnormalities	Causes	Red cell abnormalities	Causes
Normal		Spherocyte	Hereditary spherocytosis, autoimmune haemolytic anaemia, septicaemia
Macrocyte	Liver disease, alcoholism. Oval in megaloblastic anaemia	Fragments	DIC, microangiopathy, HUS, TTP, burns, cardiac valves
Target cell	Iron deficiency, liver disease, haemoglobinopathies, post-splenectomy	Elliptocyte	Hereditary elliptocytosis
Stomatocyte	Liver disease, alcoholism	Tear drop poikilocyte	Myelofibrosis, extramedullary haemopoiesis
Pencil cell	Iron deficiency	Basket cell	Oxidant damage, e.g. G6PD deficiency, unstable haemoglobin
Ecchinocyte	Liver disease, renal disease, post-splenectomy	Howell–Jolly body	Hyposplenism, post-splenectomy
Acanthocyte	Liver disease, abetalipoprotein-aemia, renal failure	Basophilic stippling	Haemoglobinopathy, lead poisoning, myelodysplasia, haemolytic anaemia
Sickle cell	Sickle cell anaemia	Malarial parasite	Malaria. Other intra-erythrocytic parasites include *Bartonella bacilliformis*, babesiosis
Microcyte	Iron deficiency, haemoglobinopathy	Siderotic granules (Pappenheimer bodies)	Disordered iron metabolism, e.g. sideroblastic anaemia, post-splenectomy

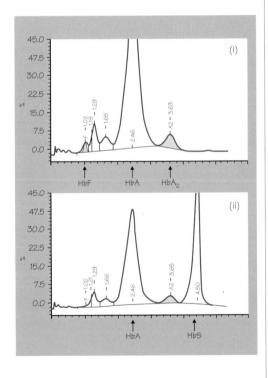

Anaemia

Anaemia is defined as a subnormal haemoglobin concentration. It is usually accompanied by a reduction in red cell count and haematocrit. The normal ranges (Appendix II) differ according to age and sex. Anaemia is not, by itself, a sufficient diagnosis; further assessment must be undertaken to establish the cause before treatment can be commenced (Table 10.1). This is done by clinical assessment (history, physical examination) and appropriate use of special investigations. A classification of anaemia according to whether red cells are large (macrocytic, normocytic) or small (microcytic) is given in Table 10.2 and further details on the specific types of anaemia are given in the appropriate chapters.

The full blood count (FBC) must be performed as an initial investigation using an automatic cell counter (Fig. 10a). The red cell indices (mean corpuscular volume, MCV; mean corpuscular haemoglobin, MCH; mean corpuscular haemoglobin concentration, MCHC; red cell distribution width, RDW) and red cell count (RBC $\times 10^{12}$/L) will give indicators of the type of anaemia (e.g. microcytic or macrocytic).

Reticulocytes (Fig.10b) are immature, non-nucleated red cells which retain RNA. They may be quantified by a manual differential count of a specially stained slide and expressed as a per cent of red cells (normal = 1–3%); or counted automatically by the cell counter and expressed as an absolute number (normal range = 50–150 $\times 10^9$/L). They increase in number, providing marrow function is intact, following increased red cell loss (e.g. haemorrhage) or destruction (e.g. haemolysis) or following treatment of haematinic deficiency.

A *blood film* is made by spreading a drop of blood on a glass slide, staining with a Romanowsky stain, and examining the film microscopically initially at low power and then at higher power. Most haematology laboratories will make a blood film only if specifically requested to do so by the clinician, in patients with a known haematological disorder or in patients who have an abnormal FBC.

A stained blood film is an excellent way of examining red cell morphology as a clue to underlying pathology (Fig. 10c). The blood film also allows estimation of the white cell differential count, though this is now usually performed automatically by the cell counter. The blood film also allows examination of morphology of white cells, platelets and any circulating non-haemopoietic cells (e.g. parasites).

Haemoglobin disorders (Chapter 18) are among the most commonly inherited conditions in mankind. Haemoglobin electrophoresis is a simple technique whereby red cells are lysed to release haemoglobin, and the lysate is applied to a gel across which an electric current is applied (see Fig. 19d). High performance liquid chromatography (HPLC) is an increasingly used automated technique used in place of haemoglobin electrophoresis (Fig. 10d). These techniques allow detection of an abnormal haemoglobin; and the relative proportions of the different normal haemoglobins (Hb A, A_2, F).

Haematinic levels (i.e. serum vitamin B_{12}, folate, ferritin, iron and iron-binding capacity) are performed by analysers using immunoassay. The results may indicate the underlying cause of anaemia. Normal ranges are given in Appendix II.

Table 10.1 Classification of anaemia according to cause

Inherited – these are usually associated with reduced red cell survival (haemolytic anaemias)
    Defects of haemoglobin, e.g. sickle cell, thalassaemia
    Defects of red cell metabolism, e.g. glucose 6 phosphate dehydrogenase deficiency
    Defects of red cell membrane, e.g. hereditary spherocytosis
Acquired
    Reduced red cell production due to
        Haematinic deficiency (iron, vitamin B_{12}, folic acid, vitamin B_6)
        Marrow replacement, e.g. by tumour (leukaemia, lymphoma)
        Marrow aplasia (see Chapter 20)
    Increased red cell destruction (haemolytic anaemia)
        Immune destruction
        Red cell fragmentation syndromes
        Chemical and physical agents
        Infections
        Paroxysmal nocturnal haemoglobinuria
Systemic illnesses
    Anaemia of chronic disease
    Renal failure, liver disease, cardiac disease

Table 10.2 Classification of anaemia according to red cell size

Macrocytic (MCV > 98 fl)
    Megaloblastic
        Vitamin B_{12} or folate deficiency
    Other
        See Table 14.1

Normocytic (MCV = 78–98 fl)
    Most haemolytic anaemias
    Secondary anaemias
    Mixed cases

Microcytic (MCV < 78 fl; MCH usually also < 27 pg/L)
    Iron deficiency
    Thalassaemia (α or β)
    Other haemoglobin defects
    Anaemia of chronic disorders (some cases)
    Congenital sideroblastic anaemia (some cases)

MCH, mean cell haemoglobin; MCV, mean cell volume

11 Iron I: physiology and deficiency

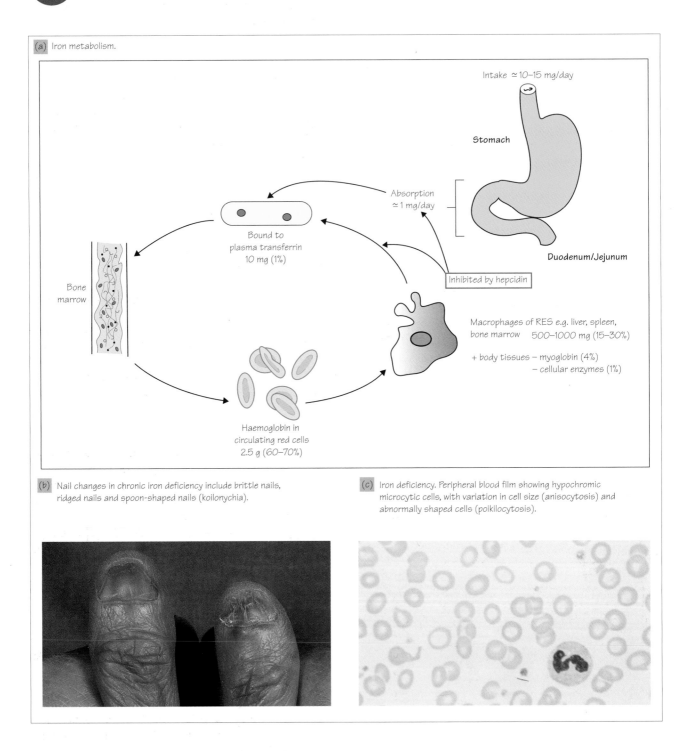

(a) Iron metabolism.

Intake ≃ 10–15 mg/day

Stomach

Absorption ≃ 1 mg/day

Duodenum/Jejunum

Bound to plasma transferrin 10 mg (1%)

Inhibited by hepcidin

Bone marrow

Macrophages of RES e.g. liver, spleen, bone marrow 500–1000 mg (15–30%)

+ body tissues – myoglobin (4%)
– cellular enzymes (1%)

Haemoglobin in circulating red cells 2.5 g (60–70%)

(b) Nail changes in chronic iron deficiency include brittle nails, ridged nails and spoon-shaped nails (koilonychia).

(c) Iron deficiency. Peripheral blood film showing hypochromic microcytic cells, with variation in cell size (anisocytosis) and abnormally shaped cells (poikilocytosis).

Distribution of body iron

Iron is contained in haemoglobin, the reticuloendothelial system (as ferritin and haemosiderin), muscle (myoglobin), plasma (bound to transferrin) and cellular enzymes (e.g. cytochromes, catalase) (Fig. 11a). Reticuloendothelial cells (macrophages) gain iron from the haemoglobin of effete red cells and release it to plasma transferrin which transports iron to bone marrow and other tissues with transferrin receptors. The iron-responsive-element-binding protein (IRE-BP) is an RNA-binding protein which binds to specific mRNA sequences and is a mechanism whereby the body's iron content regulates uptake and storage of iron by cells of the reticuloendothelial system. When iron is in excess, transferrin receptor synthesis, and therefore iron uptake, is reduced and ferritin synthesis is increased. Iron deficiency has the opposite effects.

Hepcidin

Hepcidin is a protein synthesized in the liver which controls iron absorption and circulation. It lowers cell levels of ferroportin, thus reducing both iron absorption and iron release from macrophages to transferrin. Its synthesis is controlled by various proteins, e.g. HFE, hemojuvelin, matriptase 2 and the minor transferrin receptor 2. Inflammation increases hepcidin synthesis through increased levels of IL-6. Increased iron stores stimulate hepcidin synthesis because of increased iron saturation of TFR2. Erythropoiesis lowers hepcidin synthesis because of a protein released from erythroblasts.

Iron intake, absorption and loss

The average Western diet contains 10–15 mg of iron daily, of which 5–10% (about 1 mg) is normally absorbed through the upper small intestine. Absorption is normally adjusted to body needs (increased in iron deficiency and pregnancy, reduced in iron overload). Absorption is regulated by DMT-1 at the villous tip and ferroportin at the basolateral surfaces of the enterocyte.

Iron in animal products is more easily absorbed than vegetable iron; inorganic iron in ferrous form is absorbed more than ferric form. Vitamin C enhances absorption; phytates inhibit it. Dietary intake makes up for daily loss (about 1 mg) in hair, skin, urine, faeces and menstrual blood loss in women. Infants, children and pregnant women need extra iron to expand their red cell mass and, in pregnancy, for transfer to the foetus.

Iron deficiency

Causes (Table 11.1)

• Blood loss (500 mL of normal blood contains 200–250 mg iron) – the dominant cause in Western countries.

Table 11.1 Causes of iron deficiency

Chronic blood loss
Uterine, e.g. menorrhagia or postmenopausal bleeding
Gastrointestinal, e.g. oesophageal varices, hiatus hernia, atrophic gastritis, *Helicobacter* infection, peptic ulcer, ingestion of aspirin (or other non-steroidal anti-inflammatory drugs), gastrectomy, carcinoma (stomach, caecum, colon or rectum), hookworm, angiodysplasia, colitis, diverticulosis, piles
Rarely, haematuria, haemoglobinuria, pulmonary haemosiderosis, self-inflicted blood loss

Increased demands
Prematurity
Growth*
Pregnancy*

Malabsorption
Postgastrectomy, gluten-induced enteropathy

Poor diet
Rarely the sole cause in developed countries

---

*Deficiency occurs if these are associated with poor diet

• Malabsorption – rarely a main cause.
• Poor dietary intake – a contributory cause, especially in children, menstruating females or pregnancy; a major factor in developing countries.

Clinical features

• General features of anaemia (see Chapter 10).
• Special features (minority of patients): koilonychia (Fig. 11b) or ridged brittle nails, glossitis, angular cheilosis (sore corners of mouth), pica (abnormal appetite), hair thinning and pharyngeal web formation (Paterson–Kelly syndrome).
• Features resulting from an underlying cause.
  NB: Iron deficiency is the most common cause of anaemia in all countries of the world.

Laboratory findings

• Hypochromic microcytic anaemia.
• Raised platelet count.
• Blood film appearances (Fig. 11c) include hypochromic/microcytic cells, aniso/poikilocytosis, target cells and 'pencil' cells.
• Bone marrow – not needed for diagnosis: erythroblasts show ragged irregular cytoplasm; absence of iron from stores and erythroblasts.
• Serum ferritin reduced, serum iron low with raised transferrin and raised unsaturated iron-binding capacity.

Other investigations

• History (especially for blood loss, diet, malabsorption). Tests for cause (especially in males and postmenopausal females) include occult blood tests, upper and lower gastrointestinal endoscopy, capsule (camera) endoscopy tests for hookworm, malabsorption and urine haemosiderin.
• Haemoglobin electrophoresis and/or globin gene DNA analysis to exclude thalassaemia trait or other haemoglobin defects causing a microcytic, hypochromic blood picture.

Treatment

• Oral iron – ferrous sulphate is best (200 mg, 67 mg iron per tablet) before meals three times daily.
• A reticulocyte response begins in 7 days, but treatment should be continued for 4–6 months to replenish stores.
• Side effects (e.g. abdominal pain, diarrhoea or constipation) require a lower dose, taking iron with food, or a different preparation (e.g. ferrous gluconate 300 mg, 37 mg iron per tablet).
• Poor response may be due to continued bleeding, incorrect diagnosis, malabsorption or poor compliance.
• Oral iron, often combined with folic acid, is given for iron deficiency in pregnancy.
• Intramuscular or intravenous iron is used in patients with malabsorption or who are unable to take oral iron. Intravenous iron, e.g. iron sucrose (Venofer) or iron-dextran (Cosmofer), is useful to replenish iron stores and in renal dialysis patients receiving erythropoietin therapy.

12 Iron II: overload and sideroblastic anaemia

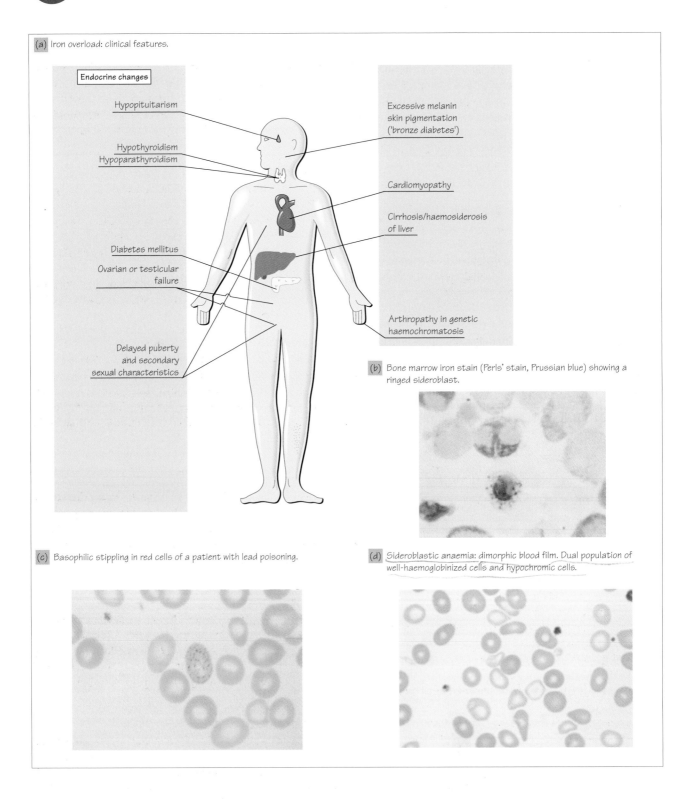

(a) Iron overload: clinical features.

Endocrine changes

Hypopituitarism

Hypothyroidism
Hypoparathyroidism

Diabetes mellitus

Ovarian or testicular
failure

Delayed puberty
and secondary
sexual characteristics

Excessive melanin
skin pigmentation
('bronze diabetes')

Cardiomyopathy

Cirrhosis/haemosiderosis
of liver

Arthropathy in genetic
haemochromatosis

(b) Bone marrow iron stain (Perls' stain, Prussian blue) showing a ringed sideroblast.

(c) Basophilic stippling in red cells of a patient with lead poisoning.

(d) Sideroblastic anaemia: dimorphic blood film. Dual population of well-haemoglobinized cells and hypochromic cells.

Iron overload

Iron overload is the pathological state in which total body stores of iron are increased, often with organ dysfunction as a result of iron deposition.

Causes
- Primary (genetic) haemochromatosis (GH) is an autosomal recessive condition associated with excessive iron absorption. Ninety per cent of cases are homozygous for a mutation in the *HFE* gene situated close to the human leucocyte antigen complex on chromosome 6. Rarely, GH is due to mutation of the hepcidin or hemojuvelin genes. All cases show low serum levels of hepcidin.
- African iron overload; dietary and genetic components.
- Excess dietary iron.
- Ineffective erythropoiesis with increased iron absorption (e.g. thalassaemia intermedia) due to inappropriately low levels of hepcidin.
- Repeated blood transfusions in patients with severe refractory anaemia, e.g. thalassaemia major, myelodysplasia. Each unit of blood contains 250 mg iron.

Clinical features
- These are mainly caused by organ dysfunction as a result of iron deposition (Fig. 12a).
- Cardiomyopathy gives rise to dysrhythmias and congestive heart failure, major cause of death.
- Growth/sexual development is reduced in children; delayed puberty, diabetes mellitus, hypothyroidism and hypoparathyroidism are frequent.
- The liver may show haemosiderosis or cirrhosis. The liver abnormality in transfusional iron overload is, however, often a result of hepatitis B or C infection.
- Excessive melanin skin pigmentation.
- Excessive infections.
- Arthropathy in genetic haemochromatosis caused by pyrophosphate deposition.

Laboratory features
- Raised serum iron and transferrin saturation.
- Raised serum ferritin.
- Increased iron in liver (histology or chemical estimation).
- Abnormal liver function tests.
- Increased urinary iron excretion in response to iron chelator therapy.
- Cardiomyopathy causes abnormal echocardiographic findings.
- MRI can detect increased iron in heart and liver.
- Endocrine abnormalities, e.g. raised blood glucose.

Treatment
- Genetic haemochromatosis: regular venesections to reduce iron level to normal, assessed by serum ferritin, serum iron and total iron-binding capacity and by liver biopsy or MRI.

- Transfusional iron overload: iron chelation is described in Chapter 18.

Sideroblastic anaemia
Definition
Sideroblastic anaemia is a refractory anaemia in which the marrow shows increased iron present as granules arranged in a ring around the nucleus in developing erythroblasts ('ringed sideroblasts'; Fig.12b). At least 15% of erythroblasts show this in the primary forms. A defect of haem synthesis is present.

Classification
- The most common form is primary acquired type (a type of myelodysplasia; see Chapter 25).
- An X-linked genetic defect in haem synthesis (usually due to mutation of δ-amino laevulinic acid synthase, ALA-S), a key enzyme in haem synthesis underlies most congenital forms, usually in males.
- Ringed sideroblasts may also occur with other haematological disorders and with alcohol, isoniazid therapy and lead poisoning.

Clinical and laboratory features
The congenital anaemia is sometimes mild (haemoglobin 8–10 g/dL) but may become more severe with age. Leucopenia and thrombocytopenia may occur in patients with myelodysplasia. Blood film may be dimorphic (Fig.12d). The mean corpuscular volume is usually raised in acquired and low in the inherited variety.

Treatment
Usually symptomatic. Regular blood transfusion and iron chelation is often required. Patients with inherited forms may respond to pyridoxine (vitamin B_6), a co-factor for ALA-S. Lenalidomide is active in acquired forms, particularly in patients who also have the 5q-chromosome abnormality.

Lead poisoning
Clinically, this presents with abdominal pain, constipation, anaemia, peripheral neuropathy and a blue (lead) line of the gums. The blood film shows punctate basophilia (blue staining dots as a result of undegraded RNA) (Fig. 12c) and features of haemolysis. The marrow may show ringed sideroblasts.

Acute iron poisoning
This is commonest in childhood and is usually accidental. Clinical features include nausea, abdominal pain, diarrhoea, gastrointestinal bleeding and abnormalities of liver function. Immediate treatment is with gastric lavage (within 1–2 hours); whole bowel irrigation may be indicated. Intravenous desferrioxamine is valuable in chelating iron and reducing risk of liver damage.

13 Megaloblastic anaemia I: vitamin B₁₂ and folic acid deficiency – biochemical basis, causes

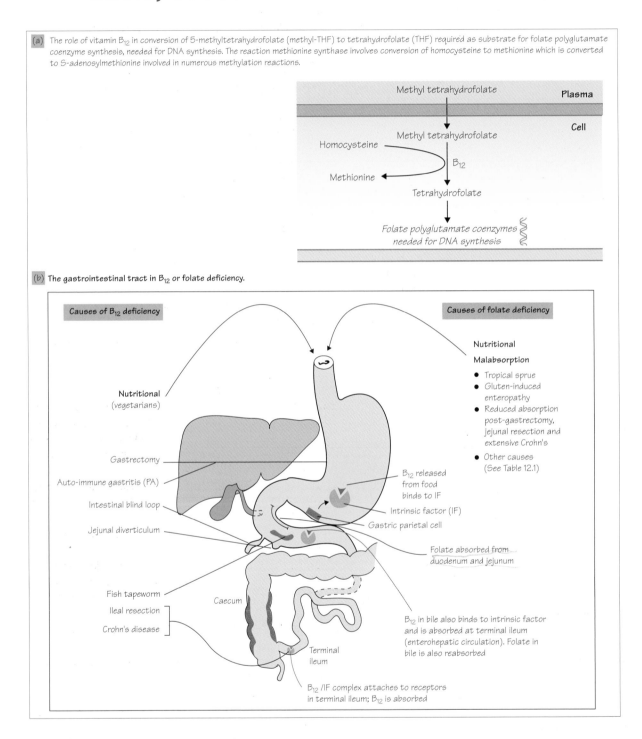

(a) The role of vitamin B_{12} in conversion of 5-methyltetrahydrofolate (methyl-THF) to tetrahydrofolate (THF) required as substrate for folate polyglutamate coenzyme synthesis, needed for DNA synthesis. The reaction methionine synthase involves conversion of homocysteine to methionine which is converted to S-adenosylmethionine involved in numerous methylation reactions.

Methyl tetrahydrofolate

Plasma

Cell

Methyl tetrahydrofolate

Homocysteine

Methionine

B_{12}

Tetrahydrofolate

Folate polyglutamate coenzymes needed for DNA synthesis

(b) The gastrointestinal tract in B_{12} or folate deficiency.

Causes of B_{12} deficiency

Causes of folate deficiency

Nutritional

Malabsorption

- Tropical sprue
- Gluten-induced enteropathy
- Reduced absorption post-gastrectomy, jejunal resection and extensive Crohn's
- Other causes (See Table 12.1)

Nutritional (vegetarians)

Gastrectomy

Auto-immune gastritis (PA)

Intestinal blind loop

Jejunal diverticulum

B_{12} released from food binds to IF

Intrinsic factor (IF)

Gastric parietal cell

Folate absorbed from duodenum and jejunum

Fish tapeworm

Ileal resection

Crohn's disease

Caecum

Terminal ileum

B_{12} in bile also binds to intrinsic factor and is absorbed at terminal ileum (enterohepatic circulation). Folate in bile is also reabsorbed

B_{12}/IF complex attaches to receptors in terminal ileum; B_{12} is absorbed

Megaloblastic anaemia is associated with an abnormal appearance of the bone marrow erythroblasts in which nuclear development is delayed and nuclear chromatin has a lacy open appearance. There is a defect in DNA synthesis usually caused by deficiency of vitamin B₁₂ (cobalamin) or folate.

Biochemical basis

Folate is an essential coenzyme for the synthesis of thymidine monophosphate (TMP) and therefore of DNA since thymine is one of the four bases needed to form DNA. B₁₂ is a coenzyme for methionine synthase, a reaction needed in the demethylation of the form of folate, 5-methyltetrahydrofolate (methyl THF), which enters the cells from plasma. The demethylation provides THF which acts as substrate for synthesis of intracellular folate polyglutamates, the coenzyme forms of folate needed in cells for DNA synthesis. During DNA synthesis, folates are oxidized to the dihydrofolate form, and the enzyme dihydrofolate reductase (inhibited by methotrexate) is required to restore them to the active THF state.

B_{12} physiology (Fig.13a)

- Adult daily requirement for B_{12} is 1 µg (normal mixed diet contains 10–15 µg). B_{12} is present only in foods of animal origin: meat, fish, eggs, milk and butter; it is absent from vegetables, cereals and fruit, unless these are contaminated by microorganisms. Normal body stores of B_{12}, largely in the liver with an enterohepatic circulation, are sufficient to last for 2–4 years.
- Dietary B_{12} after release from food and gastric 'R' binder (see below) combines with intrinsic factor (IF) secreted by gastric parietal cells (GPC). IF–B_{12} complex attaches to ileal receptors and B_{12} is absorbed.
- Absorbed B_{12} attaches to transcobalamin (TC) II which carries B_{12} in plasma to the liver, bone marrow, brain and other tissues. Most B_{12} in plasma is attached to a second B_{12}-binding protein, TC I, and is functionally inactive. TC I is synthesized by granulocytes and their precursors. Similar glycoproteins ('R' proteins or haptocorrins) occur in saliva, gastric juice and milk.
- Passive absorption (about 0.1% of oral B_{12}) occurs through buccal, gastric and duodenal mucosae.

Causes of B_{12} deficiency (Fig. 13b)

Inadequate diet

Vegans may develop B_{12} deficiency, although the intact entero-hepatic circulation of a few micrograms of B_{12} daily delays its onset. Infants born to B_{12}-deficient mothers and breast-fed by them may present with failure to thrive and megaloblastic anaemia resulting from B_{12} deficiency.

Malabsorption

Gastric causes
- Pernicious anaemia (PA) is characterized by an autoimmune gastritis, and reduced gastric secretion of IF and acid. It is often associated with other organ-specific autoimmune diseases (e.g. myxoedema, thyrotoxicosis, vitiligo, Addison's disease and hypoparathyroidism). Antibodies to IF and gastric parietal cells occur in serum (50 and 90%, respectively) of patients. PA is also associated with early greying of hair, blue eyes, blood group A, a family history of PA or related autoimmune disease and a two-to threefold increased incidence of carcinoma of the stomach. It occurs in all races and has a female/male incidence of 1.6:1. Peak age of incidence is 60 years.
- Gastrectomy (total or subtotal) leads to B_{12} deficiency.
- Congenital IF deficiency or abnormality is rare.

Intestinal causes

These include bacterial (rarely fish tapeworm) colonization of small intestine, stagnant loop syndromes, congenital and acquired defects of the ileum (e.g. ileal resection, Crohn's disease). Congenital B_{12} malabsorption with proteinuria (due to a

Table 13.1 Causes of folate deficiency

Nutritional
Especially old age, institutions, poverty, famine

Malabsorption
Gluten-induced enteropathy, dermatitis herpetiformis, tropical sprue

Excess utilization
Physiological
Pregnancy and lactation, prematurity
Pathological
Haematological diseases: haemolytic anaemias, myelofibrosis
Malignant diseases: carcinoma, lymphoma, myeloma
Inflammatory diseases: Crohn's disease, rheumatoid arthritis, extensive psoriasis, exfoliative dermatitis, malaria

Excess urinary folate loss
Congestive heart failure, chronic dialysis

Drugs
Anticonvulsants, sulphasalazine

Mixed
Liver disease, alcoholism (spirit drinkers)

genetic defect of the ileal receptor) is rare. Less severe malabsorption of food B_{12} may occur with (simple) atrophic gastritis, *Helicobacter* infection, gluten-induced enteropathy and drugs, e.g. metformin.

Folate physiology

Folates consist of a large number of compounds derived from the parent compound pteroylglutamic (folic) acid by reduction, addition of single carbon groups, e.g. methyl or formyl, and, in cells, addition of extra glutamate moieties usually four, five or six to form polyglutamates.
- Occur in most foods, especially liver and green vegetables. Normal daily diet contains 200–250 µg, of which about 50% is absorbed.
- Daily adult requirements are about 100 µg; body stores are sufficient for 4 months.
- Absorbed through the upper small intestine with conversion of all natural forms to 5-methyl tetrahydrofolate (methyl THF). A specific protein is needed for absorption of all forms of folate.

Causes of folate deficiency (Table 13.1, Fig. 13b)

- The most common cause is poor dietary intake, either alone or in association with increased folate utilization (e.g. pregnancy or haemolytic anaemia).
- Malabsorption occurs in gluten-induced enteropathy or tropical sprue.
- Increased utilization: increased cell turnover and DNA synthesis causes
- breakdown of folates; the most common causes include pregnancy, haemolytic anaemia, severe chronic inflammatory and malignant diseases and anticonvulsant drugs.
- Folate is loosely bound to protein in plasma and is easily removed by dialysis.

14 Megaloblastic anaemia II: clinical features, treatment and other macrocytic anaemias

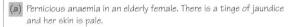

(a) Pernicious anaemia in an elderly female. There is a tinge of jaundice and her skin is pale.

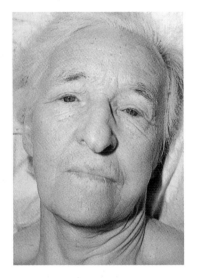

(b) Peripheral blood in megaloblastic anaemia, showing a hypersegmented neutrophil (A), oval macrocytes and poikilocytosis (variation in red cell shape).

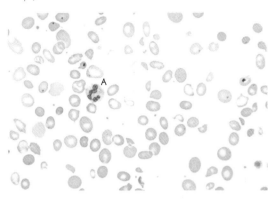

(c) (i) Bone marrow in megaloblastic anaemia showing megaloblasts. These are nucleated erythroid cells with open lacy chromatin and delayed nuclear maturation. (ii) Megaloblasts with developing myeloid cells; the cell with a C-shaped nucleus (arrow) is a giant metamyelocyte.

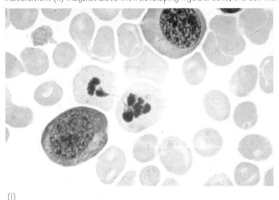

(i)

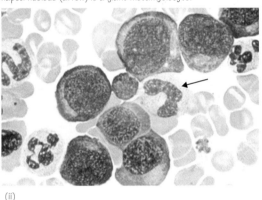

(ii)

B₁₂ deficiency

Clinical features

- Gradual onset of features of anaemia.
- Mild jaundice, caused by ineffective erythropoiesis.
- Glossitis (Fig. 14a) and angular cheilosis and, if severe, sterility (either sex) and reversible melanin skin pigmentation.
- B_{12} deficiency causes a symmetrical neuropathy affecting the pyramidal tracts and posterior columns of the spinal cord (subacute combined degeneration of the cord) and the peripheral nerves. Patients present with tingling in the feet (more than the hands), difficulty in gait, visual or psychiatric disorders.

- B_{12} or folate deficiency is associated with increased plasma homocysteine and, in pregnancy, with an increased incidence of foetal neural tube defects.
- Patients may be asymptomatic and detected by a routine blood test.

Laboratory findings

- Macrocytic anaemia with oval macrocytes and hypersegmented neutrophils (more than five nuclear lobes) (Fig. 14b).
- Moderate reduction in leucocyte and platelet counts (severe cases).

- Biochemical tests show raised serum bilirubin (indirect), lactate dehydrogenase.
- In B_{12} deficiency, the serum B_{12} is low, serum folate is normal or raised and red cell folate is normal or low.
- Bone marrow is hypercellular, increased proportion of early cells, megaloblastic erythropoiesis and giant metamyelocytes (Fig. 14c).
- Raised serum methylmalonic acid (B_{12} deficiency), raised serum homocysteine (either B_{12} or folate deficiency).

Tests for causes of B_{12} deficiency

These include history (diet, previous surgery), tests for intrinsic factor (IF) and parietal cell antibodies, upper gastrointestinal endoscopy and radioactive B_{12} absorption studies. These distinguish gastric from intestinal causes of B_{12} malabsorption. The amount of radioactive B_{12} absorbed is measured in a 24-hour urine sample after an oral radioactive dose given with a 'flushing' dose of 1 mg unlabelled B_{12}. The test can be repeated (Part II) with the labelled B_{12} given with IF. B_{12} absorption is low and corrected by IF in pernicious anaemia but is low and not corrected by IF in intestinal diseases.

Treatment

Treatment of B_{12} deficiency is 1 mg hydroxocobalamin intramuscularly, repeated every 2–3 days until six injections have been given; then one injection every 3 months for life unless the cause of deficiency has been corrected.

Folate deficiency

The clinical features of folate deficiency are the same as B_{12} deficiency, but folate deficiency does not cause a similar neuropathy. Folic acid therapy in early pregnancy reduces the incidence of neural tube defects (NTD) (anencephaly, spina bifida, encephalocoele) in the foetus.

Tests for causes of deficiency

These include history (diet, previous surgery, drug therapy, alcohol, other associated diseases), antitransglutaminase and endomysial antibodies, and tests for malabsorption (e.g. duodenal biopsy). The serum folate is low, red cell folate low and serum B_{12} is normal or slightly reduced.

Treatment

Treatment is 5-mg folic acid daily for 4 months, then decide whether to continue folic acid, e.g. 5-mg folic acid once weekly or 400 µg daily indefinitely. Folate therapy corrects the anaemia but not the neuropathy of B_{12} deficiency. Indeed, administration

Table 14.1 Causes of raised mean corpuscular volume other than megaloblastic anaemia

1	Alcohol
2	Liver disease
3	Myxoedema
4	Reticulocytosis
5	Cytotoxic drugs
6	Aplastic anaemia
7	Pregnancy
8	Myelodysplastic syndromes
9	Myeloma
10	Neonatal

of folic acid to a severely B_{12}-deficient individual may precipitate or worsen B_{12} neuropathy. Pregnant women are given folic acid 400 µg daily to reduce the incidence of megaloblastic anaemia and neural tube defects in the foetus. Dietary fortification with folate is used in the USA and many countries (not UK) to reduce incidence of NTD. It may also reduce the incidence of cardiovascular diseases and stroke by lowering homocysteine levels, but this is not established.

Other causes of megaloblastic anaemia

Defects of B_{12} or folate metabolism include congenital transcobalamin (TC) II deficiency which leads to B_{12} malabsorption and failure of B_{12} to enter cells resulting in megaloblastic anaemia (MA) in early infancy. N_2O anaesthesia reversibly inactivates body B_{12}, and prolonged or repeated exposure may cause megaloblastic anaemia or B_{12} neuropathy. Antifolate drugs include the inhibitors of dihydrofolate reductase (methotrexate, pyrimethamine and trimethoprim) which have progressively less activity against the human compared to the bacterial enzyme. Folinic acid (5-formyl-THF) is used to overcome methotrexate or cotrimoxale toxicity. Megaloblastic anaemia also occurs with cytotoxic drug therapy (e.g. 6-mercaptopurine, cytosine arabinoside or hydroxycarbamide) or, rarely, inborn errors, e.g. orotic aciduria.

Causes of macrocytosis

Alcohol is the most frequent cause. The haemoglobin level is usually normal. Mean corpuscular volume is not usually as high as in severe MA. White cell and platelet counts are normal in alcohol or other conditions (see Table 14.1) unless the underlying marrow disease affects these. Other distinguishing features are that the red cells are circular rather than oval, hypersegmented neutrophils are absent and the marrow is normoblastic.

15 Haemolytic anaemias I: general

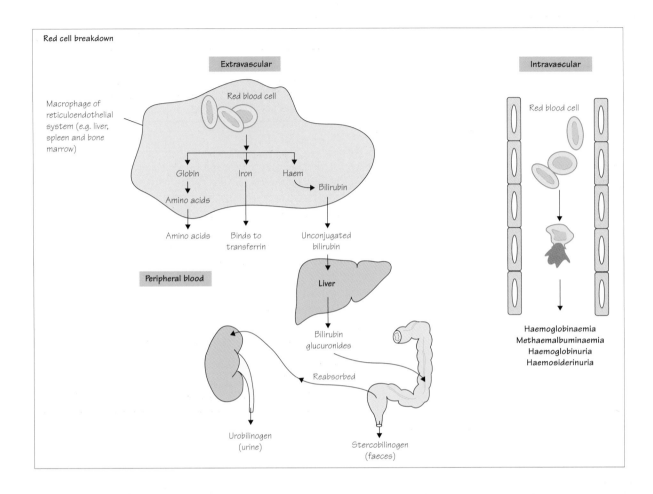

Haemolytic anaemias I: general

Haemolytic anaemias are caused by a shortened red cell lifespan; the normal mean red cell life (MRCL) is 120 days. Red cell production can be increased 6–8 times by normal bone marrow and haemolytic anaemia (HA) occurs if MRCL falls to 15 days or less, particularly in the presence of ineffective erythropoiesis, haematinic deficiency or marrow disease. Haemolysis may be caused by a fault in the red cell, usually inherited, or an abnormality in its environment, usually acquired (Table 15.1).

Physiology of red cell destruction

(Fig. 15)

Red cell destruction is normally extravascular in the macrophages of the reticuloendothelial system, bone marrow, liver and spleen. Globin is degraded to amino acids, haem to protoporphyrin, carbon monoxide and iron. Protoporphyrin is metabolized to bilirubin, conjugated to a glucuronide in the liver, excreted in faeces (as stercobilinogen) and, after reabsorption, urine as urobilinogen. Iron is recycled to plasma and combined to transferrin. Some iron remains in the macrophages as ferritin and haemosiderin. Haptoglobins are plasma proteins which bind haemoglobin to form a complex which is removed by the liver; their level is reduced in haemolysis as well as in liver disease. Pathological red cell destruction is also usually extravascular. However, it may be intravascular (Table 15.2). Some haemoglobin may then appear in plasma, where it is toxic and may cause fever, rigours and tissue damage. It is then excreted unchanged in the urine and may cause renal damage; it is also partly reabsorbed by the renal tubules and broken down to haemosiderin.

Clinical features

- Anaemia (unless fully compensated haemolysis).
- Jaundice (usually mild) caused by unconjugated bilirubin in plasma; bilirubin is absent from the urine.
- An increased incidence of pigment (bilirubin) gallstones.
- Splenomegaly – in many types.
- Ankle ulcers, especially sickle cell anaemia, thalassaemia intermedia and hereditary spherocytosis.
- Expansion of marrow with, in children, bone expansion, e.g. frontal bossing in β-thalassaemia major.

Table 15.1 Classification of haemolytic anaemia

Hereditary	Acquired
Membrane Hereditary spherocytosis, hereditary elliptocytosis South-East Asian ovalocytosis	**Immune** *Autoimmune* Warm antibody type Idiopathic or secondary to SLE, CLL, drugs, e.g. methyldopa Cold antibody type Idiopathic or secondary to infections (e.g. mycoplasma, infectious mononucleosis), lymphoma, paroxysmal cold haemoglobinuria
Metabolism G6PD deficiency Pyruvate kinase deficiency Other rare enzyme deficiencies	*Alloimmune* Haemolytic transfusion reactions Haemolytic disease of newborn
Haemoglobin Haemoglobin defect (Hb S, Hb C, unstable) (see Chapter 19)	**Red cell fragmentation syndromes** Cardiac valve, 'march' haemoglobinuria *Microangiopathic haemolytic anaemia* Thrombotic thrombocytopenia purpura Haemolytic uraemic syndrome Disseminated intravascular coagulation
	Infections e.g. malaria, clostridia
	Chemical and physical agents e.g. drugs, industrial/domestic substances, burns
	Secondary e.g. liver and renal disease
	Paroxysmal nocturnal haemoglobinuria

CLL, chronic lymphocytic leukaemia; SLE, systemic lupus erythematosus

Table 15.2 Causes of intravascular haemolysis

Mismatched blood transfusion (usually ABO)
G6PD deficiency with oxidant stress
Red cell fragmentation syndromes
Some autoimmune haemolytic anaemias
Some drug- and infection-induced haemolytic anaemias
Paroxysmal nocturnal haemoglobinuria
March haemoglobinuria
Unstable haemoglobin

- Aplastic crises caused by parvovirus infection.
- Megaloblastic anaemia caused by folate deficiency.

Laboratory features

- Haemoglobin level may be normal or reduced.
- Raised reticulocyte count.
- Blood film may show polychromasia (blue staining in young red cells), altered red cell shape, e.g. spherocytes, elliptocytes, sickle cells or fragmented cells.
- Bone marrow shows increased erythropoiesis.
- Serum indirect (unconjugated) bilirubin is raised.
- Serum haptoglobins absent.
- Intravascular haemolysis leads to raised plasma and urine haemoglobin, positive serum (Schumm's) test for methaemalbumin, urine haemosiderin.

Haemolytic anaemias II: inherited membrane and enzyme defects

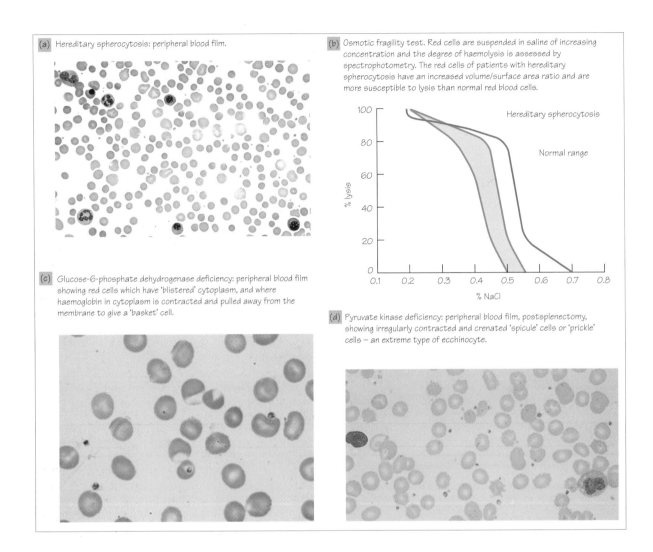

(a) Hereditary spherocytosis: peripheral blood film.

(b) Osmotic fragility test. Red cells are suspended in saline of increasing concentration and the degree of haemolysis is assessed by spectrophotometry. The red cells of patients with hereditary spherocytosis have an increased volume/surface area ratio and are more susceptible to lysis than normal red blood cells.

(c) Glucose-6-phosphate dehydrogenase deficiency: peripheral blood film showing red cells which have 'blistered' cytoplasm, and where haemoglobin in cytoplasm is contracted and pulled away from the membrane to give a 'basket' cell.

(d) Pyruvate kinase deficiency: peripheral blood film, postsplenectomy, showing irregularly contracted and crenated 'spicule' cells or 'prickle' cells — an extreme type of ecchinocyte.

Membrane abnormalities
Hereditary spherocytosis

This is the most common inherited haemolytic anaemia (HA) in white people. It is autosomal dominant with variable severity and may present as severe neonatal HA, as symptomatic HA later in life or may be an incidental finding. Defect is in a red cell membrane protein, e.g. ankyrin, band 3; 25% of cases are new mutations. Affected red cells lose membrane during passage through the reticuloendothelial system, especially the spleen. The cells become progressively more spherical (decreased surface area/volume ratio) and microcytic. They are destroyed prematurely, mainly in the spleen. Hereditary elliptocytosis (HE) is a similar, usually milder, abnormality.

Clinical features

Clinical features are those generally associated with HA. The spleen is usually enlarged.

Laboratory features

• Blood film: microspherocytes and polychromasia (Fig. 16a).
• Haemoglobin level variable.
• Tests for HA are positive (see Chapter 15).
• Special tests: osmotic fragility increased (Fig. 16b), N-ethylmaleimide test for band 3 abnormality, autohaemolysis increased and corrected by addition of glucose.
• Direct antiglobulin test is negative (excluding warm autoimmune HA which can cause a similar blood film appearance).

Treatment

• Splenectomy corrects the decrease in lifespan, although spherocytosis persists; may not be needed in mild cases; defer if possible in children until over the age of 6 years.
• Give folic acid prophylactically for severe cases.

- Pigment gallstones may cause cholecystitis.
- If cholecystectomy required, perform splenectomy also to reduce risk of recurrent gallstones.

South-East Asian ovalocytosis
This is an inherited red cell membrane protein defect (band 3), in which carriers have a degree of protection against malaria.

Enzyme abnormalities
Glucose-6-phosphate dehydrogenase deficiency
Glucose-6-phosphate dehydrogenase (G6PD) is the first enzyme in the hexose monophosphate pathway (see Fig. 2d) which generates reducing power as reduced nicotinamide adenine dinucleotide phosphate (NADPH). Deficiency results in red cells being susceptible to oxidant stress. The gene is on the X chromosome so inheritance is sex-linked. Males are typically affected, though females may show mild abnormalities. Many different DNA mutations within the gene give rise to mutant enzymes which are unstable and have reduced activity. Affected males develop HA when the red cells are exposed to oxidant stress, especially by drugs, infections, ingestion of fava beans (a type of broad bean) and during the neonatal period (Table 16.1). Infection is associated with increased production of oxidants (e.g. H_2O_2 from neutrophils). G6PD deficiency is one of the commonest of all inherited disorders and is common in black, Mediterranean, Middle Eastern and oriental populations. Individuals with G6PD deficiency have a degree of protection against malaria.

Clinical and laboratory features
- Blood count and film normal between crises.
- During crises features of acute intravascular haemolysis; renal failure may occur in severe episodes.
- Blood film in a crisis (see Fig. 16c) shows red cells with absent haemoglobin ('bite' and 'blister' cells) and polychromasia. Heinz bodies (denatured haemoglobin) may be seen in a reticulocyte preparation with supravital staining.
- Haemolysis is usually self-limited because of the increased G6PD activity in reticulocytes.
- Chronic non-spherocytic HA (CNSHA) occurs rarely with certain mutant enzymes.

Table 16.1 Agents which may cause haemolytic anaemia in G6PD deficiency

Infections and other acute illnesses, e.g. diabetic ketoacidosis

Drugs
 Antimalarials, e.g. primaquine
 Sulphonamides and sulphones, e.g. cotrimoxazole, sulphanilamide, dapsone, salazopyrine

 Other antibacterial agents, e.g. nitrofurans, chloramphenicol
 Analgesics, e.g. aspirin (moderate doses are safe)
 Antihelminths, e.g. β-naphthol, stibophen, niridazole
 Miscellaneous, e.g. vitamin K analogues, naphthalene (mothballs), probenecid

Fava beans (broad beans)

- Neonatal jaundice is frequent.
- Screening tests for red cell G6PD deficiency measure the generation of NADPH. The enzyme may also be characterized by electrophoresis, assay of activity and DNA analysis. Diagnosis should, when possible, be undertaken in the steady state as reticulocytes generally have higher enzyme activity and the raised reticulocyte count following haemolysis may lead to a false normal result.

Management
- Stop offending drugs or fava bean ingestion.
- Treat infection if present.
- Transfuse red cells if necessary.
- Splenectomy may ameliorate HA in rare CNSHA.

Pyruvate kinase deficiency
Pyruvate kinase (PK) deficiency is the most frequent enzyme deficiency in the Embden–Meyerhof (glycolytic) pathway to cause CNSHA (see Fig. 16d). Inheritance is autosomal recessive. The O_2-dissociation curve is shifted to the right, so symptoms are mild in comparison to the degree of anaemia. Splenectomy partly improves the anaemia.

Other enzyme deficiencies are rare causes of CNSHA and are frequently associated with musculoskeletal disease.

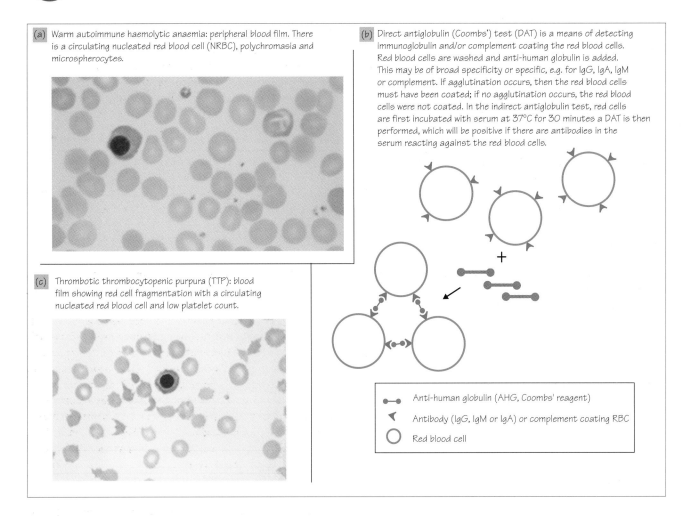

(a) Warm autoimmune haemolytic anaemia: peripheral blood film. There is a circulating nucleated red blood cell (NRBC), polychromasia and microspherocytes.

(b) Direct antiglobulin (Coombs') test (DAT) is a means of detecting immunoglobulin and/or complement coating the red blood cells. Red blood cells are washed and anti-human globulin is added. This may be of broad specificity or specific, e.g. for IgG, IgA, IgM or complement. If agglutination occurs, then the red blood cells must have been coated; if no agglutination occurs, the red blood cells were not coated. In the indirect antiglobulin test, red cells are first incubated with serum at 37°C for 30 minutes a DAT is then performed, which will be positive if there are antibodies in the serum reacting against the red blood cells.

(c) Thrombotic thrombocytopenic purpura (TTP): blood film showing red cell fragmentation with a circulating nucleated red blood cell and low platelet count.

Anti-human globulin (AHG, Coombs' reagent)

Antibody (IgG, IgM or IgA) or complement coating RBC

Red blood cell

Autoimmune haemolytic anaemia

This is caused by autoantibodies against the red cell membrane. It is divided into warm and cold antibody types and each may be idiopathic or secondary to other diseases (see Table 15.1).

Warm autoimmune haemolytic anaemia

Antibody, typically IgG, has maximum activity at 37°C.

Clinical and laboratory features

• Presents at any age, in either sex, with features of extravascular haemolytic anaemia of varying severity.
• The spleen is often enlarged.
• Blood film shows microspherocytes, polychromasia, ± circulating nucleated red blood cells (Fig. 17a).
• Direct antiglobulin test (DAT) is positive (Fig. 17b).
• Antibody may be non-specific or directed against antigens in the Rh system.
• IgG or IgG + complement (C3d) is detected on the red cell.
• Free antibody may be present in the serum.

• May be associated with immune thrombocytopenia (Evans syndrome).
• Antibody-coated red cells are destroyed in the reticuloendothelial system, especially the spleen.

Treatment

• Corticosteroids, e.g. prednisolone 1 mg/kg orally with subsequent gradual reduction.
• Blood transfusion, if necessary.
• Consider splenectomy if steroid therapy fails.
• Other immunosuppressive drugs, e.g. azathioprine, cyclosporin, cyclophosphamide, mycophenolate, rituximab (anti-CD20).
• Remove cause, e.g. drug.
• Treat underlying disease, e.g. chronic lymphocytic leukaemia, systemic lupus erythematosus.

Cold autoimmune haemolytic anaemia

Antibody, typically IgM, has maximum activity at 4°C.

Clinical and laboratory features

- Raynaud's phenomenon affecting the fingers, toes, nose and ears.
- Positive DAT with C3d on red cells.
  - Haemolysis may be intravascular and if severe may cause rigours, haemoglobinuria, renal failure
- Cold agglutinins, usually IgM and directed against I or i antigen (especially in infectious mononucleosis) on red cells, are present in serum, often to titres of 1:4000 or more. In primary form (cold haemagglutinin disease), the antibody is monoclonal and the patient may ultimately develop non-Hodgkin lymphoma.
- Paroxysmal cold haemoglobinuria is a rare syndrome, precipitated by infections. Intravascular haemolysis is caused by the Donath–Landsteiner antibody which binds red cells in the cold, but causes lysis at 37°C.

Treatment

- Keep the patient warm.
- Consider immunosuppression with chlorambucil, cyclophosphamide or rituximab.
- Consider plasma exchange to lower antibody titre.

Alloimmune haemolytic anaemia

This is caused when antibody produced by one individual reacts against red cells of another. The three important situations are:
1 mismatched blood transfusions (see Chapter 47);
2 haemolytic disease of the newborn (see Chapter 45) and
3 following marrow or solid organ transplantation.

Drug-induced immune haemolytic anaemia

See Chapter 50.

Red cell fragmentation syndromes

These occur when red cells are exposed to an abnormal surface (e.g. non-endothelialized artificial heart valve or arterial graft), or flow through small vessels containing fibrin strands (e.g. in disseminated intravascular coagulation) or damaged small vessels. This is termed microangiopathic haemolytic anaemia (MAHA) and occurs in thrombotic thrombocytopenic purpura, haemolytic uraemic syndrome, widespread adenocarcinoma, malignant hypertension, pre-eclampsia and meningococcal

septicaemia. Haemolysis is both extra- and intravascular; blood film shows deeply staining fragmented red cells (see Fig. 17c).

Infections

These may cause haemolysis by:
- direct damage to red cells (e.g. malaria);
- toxin production (e.g. clostridium perfringens);
- oxidant stress in G6PD-deficient individuals;
- MAHA (e.g. meningococcal septicaemia);
- autoantibody formation (e.g. infectious mononucleosis) and
- extravascular destruction (e.g. malaria).

Chemical and physical agents

Some drugs, e.g. dapsone, or chemicals, e.g. chlorate, cause haemolysis by oxidation even with normal G6PD levels. Severe burns and snakebites may also cause haemolysis.

Paroxysmal nocturnal haemoglobinuria

This is a clonal disorder in which haemolysis is caused by a rare acquired mutation of the PIG-A gene in haemopoietic stem cells. This results in a defect of the phosphatidyl inositol anchor which tethers a large number of proteins to the cell membrane. The cells become abnormally sensitive to complement-mediated haemolysis because of lack of proteins that protect against complement, e.g. CD55 (DAF) and CD59 (MIRL). It is often associated with a hypoplastic marrow with neutropenia and thrombocytopenia. The clinical course is frequently complicated by recurrent venous thromboses, especially of large veins, e.g. hepatic or portal; also by iron deficiency and infections. Diagnosis is made by a positive acid lysis (Ham's) test and the presence of red cells lacking the CD55 or CD59 antigens.

Treatment

Iron is given for iron deficiency resulting from chronic intravascular haemolysis.
- Transfusion of leucodepleted red cells may be necessary.
- Warfarin may be needed lifelong to prevent thrombosis.
- A monoclonal antibody, eculizumab that inhibits the activation of terminal complement components by binding to C5, may be used to reduce haemolysis.
- Allogeneic stem cell transplant for serious cases in young adults.

Haemolytic anaemias IV: genetic defects of haemoglobin – thalassaemia

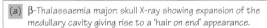

(a) β-Thalassaemia major: skull X-ray showing expansion of the medullary cavity giving rise to a 'hair on end' appearance.

(b) β-Thalassaemia major: peripheral blood film showing hypochromic microcytic red cells, target cells, poikilocytes and nucleated red blood cells. The few well-haemoglobinized cells are transfused red cells.

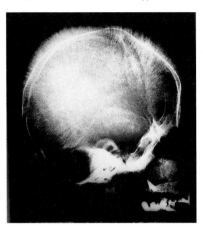

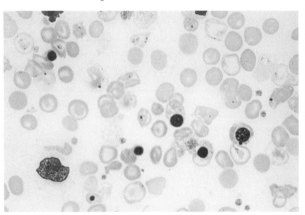

Genetic disorders of haemoglobin comprise:

1 disorders of globin chain synthesis (the thalassaemias);

2 structural defects of haemoglobin which give rise to haemolysis (e.g. sickle cell anaemia, haemoglobin C);

3 unstable haemoglobins (rare) and

4 structural disorders giving rise to polycythaemia or methaemoglobinaemia (rare).

The first and second have a wide global prevalence, particularly where malaria is, or was, common, as the carrier states give some protection against falciparum malaria. Compound heterozygote states of a thalassaemic allele and a haemoglobin structural variant allele frequently occur and include sickle/β-thalassaemia and Hb E/β-thalassaemia.

Thalassaemia

These autosomal recessive syndromes divide into α- and β-thalassaemia depending on whether there is reduced synthesis of α- or β-globin (Table 18.1).

α-Thalassaemia

Normally there are four α-globin genes, two on each chromosome 16 (see Fig. 2b). Severity of α-thalassaemia depends on the number of α-genes deleted or, less frequently, dysfunctional.

Hydrops foetalis

In hydrops foetalis all four α-genes are inactive. The foetus is unable to make either foetal ($\alpha_2\gamma_2$) or adult Hb A ($\alpha_2\beta_2$) haemoglobin. Death occurs *in utero* or neonatally.

Haemoglobin H disease

This is caused by deletion or functional inactivity of three of the four α-genes. Markedly microcytic, hypochromic anaemia (Hb 6–11.0 g/dL) with splenomegaly is usual. Bone deformities and features of iron overload do not occur. Haemoglobin

electrophoresis shows 4–10% haemoglobin H (β_4) and supravital staining shows 'golf ball' cells.

α-Thalassaemia trait

This is a one or two α-gene deletion with microcytic, hypochromic red cells with raised red cell count ($>5.5 \times 10^9$/L). Mild anaemia occurs in some cases with two α-genes deleted.

β-Thalassaemia

Thalassaemia major

Complete (β°) or almost complete (β^r) failure of β-globin chain synthesis resulting from one of over 400 different point mutations or deletions in the β-globin gene or its controlling sequences on chromosome 11. There is a severe imbalance of α:β-chains with deposition of α-chains in erythroblasts, ineffective erythropoiesis, severe anaemia and extramedullary haemopoiesis.

Clinical features

• Anaemia presents at the age of 3–6 months when the switch from γ- to β-chain synthesis normally occurs. Milder cases present later (up to the age of 4 yr).

• Failure to thrive, intercurrent infection, pallor, mild jaundice.

• Enlargement of the liver and spleen, expansion of the bones – especially of the skull – with bossing and a 'hair-on-end' appearance on X-ray (Fig. 18a); thalassaemic facies, caused by expansion of skull and facial bones.

• Features of iron overload as a result of blood transfusions and increased iron absorption include melanin pigmentation, growth/endocrine defects, e.g. diabetes mellitus, hypothyroidism, hypoparathyroidism, failure of sexual development, cardiac failure or arrhythmia, liver abnormality (see Chapter 12).

Table 18.1 Classification of thalassaemia

Clinical phenotype	Thalassaemia (thal) syndrome
Hydrops foetalis	Homozygous α-thal major → complete lack of α-globin
Thalassaemia major	Homozygous β or doubly heterozygous thal major → complete or almost complete lack of β-globin
Thalassaemia intermedia	See below
Thalassaemia trait	Heterozygous β-thalassaemia (β-thal minor, lack of one functional β-globin gene*)
	Heterozygous α-thalassaemia (α-thal minor, lack of one or two α-globin genes†)

*Normal individual has two (one from each parent on each allele)
†Normal individual has four (two from each parent on each allele)

Laboratory findings
- Severe anaemia (Hb 2–6 g/dL) with reduced mean corpuscular volume and mean corpuscular haemoglobin.
- Blood film (Fig. 18b) shows hypochromic, microcytic cells, target cells, erythroblasts and, often, myelocytes.
- Bone marrow is hypercellular with erythroid hyperplasia.
- Globin chain synthesis studies show absent, or severely deficient, β-chain synthesis. Foetal haemoglobin variably increased.
- DNA analysis reveals the specific mutations or deletions.

Management
- Regular transfusions of packed red cells to maintain haemoglobin above 9–10 g/dL, leucodepleted to reduce risk of human leukocyte antigen (HLA) sensitization and transmission of disease, e.g. cytomegalovirus.
- Iron chelation therapy has been with subcutaneous desferrioxamine (DFX) over 8–12 hours on 5–7 nights weekly. Additional DFX may be given intravenously at the time of blood transfusion via a separate bag. Oral vitamin C increases iron excretion with DFX. Side effects of DFX include hearing loss, visual defects and growth impairment. The main problem with its use is lack of compliance.

Two orally active chelators are now available in most countries. Deferiprone is given in three daily doses and is more effective than DFX at removing cardiac iron; side effects include agranulocytosis, arthralgia. Deferasirox is given once daily, is well tolerated and is increasingly used as first choice. Its cardioprotective effectiveness remains to be fully established. Iron chelation therapy is monitored clinically and by changes in serum ferritin, cardiac and liver iron measured by MRI.
- Hepatitis B is prevented by early immunization. Patients who already have chronic active hepatitis caused by hepatitis C may need α-interferon + ribavirin therapy.
- Splenectomy is necessary if blood requirements are excessively high. Defer if possible until the age of 5 years, precede by immunization (see Chapter 5) and follow by oral penicillin therapy for life. If the platelet count remains raised, low-dose aspirin reduces the risk of thromboembolism.
- Stem cell transplantation from an HLA-matching sibling may give long-term disease-free survival of up to 90% in good-risk patients, but nearer 50% in poor risk (previously poorly chelated with iron overload and liver fibrosis).
- Treat complications of iron overload: heart, endocrine organs, liver damage.
- Osteoporosis may occur as a result of marrow expansion, endocrine deficiencies.

Thalassaemia intermedia
A variable syndrome milder than thalassaemia major, with later onset, and characterized by moderately severe (Hb 6–10 g/dL), hypochromic, microcytic anaemia requiring either few or no transfusions. There is milder imbalance of α:β + γ-globin chain synthesis than in thalassaemia major. This may be due to inheritance of a milder β-chain defect, increased capacity to produce γ-chains or co-inheritance of an α-thalassaemia allele leading to reduced α-chain synthesis. Hepatosplenomegaly, extramedullary haemopoiesis, anaemia and bone deformities may occur. Iron overload occurs as a result of irregular blood transfusions and increased gastrointestinal iron absorption.

β-Thalassaemia trait
A mild hypochromic microcytic anaemia with a raised red cell count ($>5.5 \times 10^{12}$/L) and raised haemoglobin A$_2$ ($\alpha_2\delta_2$) level ($>3.5\%$). Iron stores are normal. Accurate diagnosis allows genetic counselling and avoidance of inappropriate iron therapy.

Prenatal diagnosis of haemoglobin defects
Prenatal diagnosis is available using either DNA (chorionic villous or amniotic fluid) or foetal blood. Carriers must first be identified (screening by blood count in ethnic minority groups, at preconception counselling or in the antenatal clinic). If a mother is a carrier, her partner must be tested. If both are carriers, there is a one in four chances that the foetus is homozygous or normal and a one in two chances that it is a carrier. Foetal DNA is usually amplified by use of the polymerase chain reaction and the DNA mutations are detected. If the foetus is severely affected, e.g. by thalassaemia major, the couple should be counselled and termination of pregnancy offered, if appropriate.

(a) '(a) Blood film in sickle cell disease showing a sickle cell (A), a target cell (B) and a red cell with a Howell–Jolly body (HJB) (C). HJBs are removed by spleen; adult patients with sickle cell disease have reduced spleen function.'

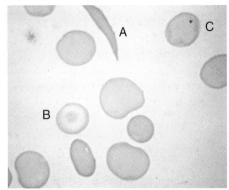

(b) Sickle cell anaemia: bony changes. X-ray showing avascular necrosis of the head of the humerus.

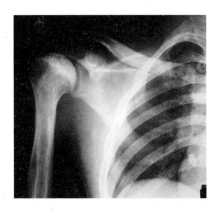

(d) Haemoglobin electrophoresis (Hb Ep). A lysate of red cells is applied to a gel and an electric current is applied. The upper panel shows migration of different haemoglobins in acid agar gel (pH 6.0) and the lower panel shows migration in cellulose acetate at alkaline pH. Haemoglobins S and F and haemoglobins A2, C and E run together on cellulose acetate and must be distinguished by acid agar Hb Ep.

(c) Sickle cell/β-thalassaemia (Hb S/β-thal): peripheral blood film. Sickle cells, target cells (arrow), hypochromasia and a low mean corpuscular volume (MCV) are characteristic.

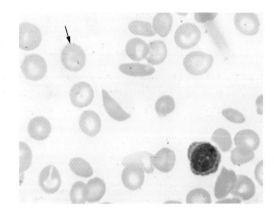

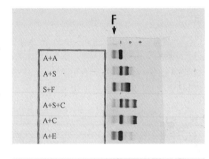

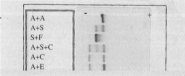

Sickle cell disease

Sickle cell disease (homozygous sickle cell anaemia) is a chronic haemolytic anaemia caused by a point mutation in the β-globin gene causing substitution of valine for glutamic acid in the sixth position of the β-globin chain. This causes insolubility of Hb S in its deoxygenated state. The insoluble chains crystallize in the red cells causing sickling (Fig. 19a) and vascular occlusion. The disease is most common in Africans (one in five West Africans are carriers – they have some protection against falciparum malaria). The mutant gene also occurs in other parts of the world where malaria is, or was, prevalent, e.g. the Middle East, Far East and the Indian subcontinent.

Clinical features

These resemble those of other chronic haemolytic anaemias, punctuated with different types of crisis.

1 Vaso-occlusive with blockage of small vessels is caused by increased sickling; common precipitants are infection, dehydration, acidosis and deoxygenation. Abdominal pain is caused by infarction affecting abdominal organs; bone pain may occur in the back, pelvis, ribs and long bones. Infarction may affect the central nervous system – causing a stroke or fits – lungs, spleen or kidneys. In children, the 'hand–foot syndrome' is caused by infarction of the metaphyses of the small bones.

2 Visceral sequestration crisis is caused by sickling with pooling of red cells in the liver, spleen or lungs. Sequestration in the lungs is partly responsible for the acute chest syndrome, though infarction and infection contribute.

3 Aplastic crisis occurs following infection by B19 parvovirus. This causes temporary arrest of erythropoiesis which in healthy individuals is of no consequence, but in patients with reduced red cell survival, such as Hb SS, can rapidly cause severe anaemia requiring blood transfusion.

- Increased susceptibility to infection. Splenic function is reduced because infarction leads to autosplenectomy. Pneumococcal infections may lead to pneumonia and meningitis. Infarction of intestinal mucosa predisposes to *Salmonella* infection and osteomyelitis may result.
- Other clinical features include pigment gallstones with cholecystitis, chronic leg ulcers, avascular necrosis of the femoral and humeral heads (Fig. 19b) or other bones, cardiomyopathy, pulmonary hypertension, proliferative retinopathy and renal papillary necrosis (leading to polyuria, failure to concentrate urine and tendency to dehydration).

Laboratory features

- Haemoglobin level is 7–9 g/dL, but symptoms of anaemia are usually mild (the O_2 dissociation curve of Hb S is shifted to the right, see Chapter 2).
- Blood film shows sickle cells, target cells and often features of splenic atrophy (see Fig. 19a).
- Screening tests for sickling demonstrate increased turbidity of the blood after deoxygenation (e.g. with dithionate or Na_2HPO_4). Haemoglobin electrophoresis (Fig. 19d) or high-performance liquid chromatography shows haemoglobin with an abnormal migration. In Hb SS, there is absence of Hb A. Hb F level is usually mildly raised (5–10%).
  - Cranial Doppler studies can reveal flow disturbances predisposing to stroke.

Treatment

- General – avoid known precipitants of sickle cell crisis, especially dehydration and infections. Give folic acid, pneumococcal, HIB and meningococcal vaccination and oral penicillin indefinitely to compensate for splenic atrophy.
- Vaso-occlusive crisis is treated with hydration, usually intravenous normal saline, analgesia (e.g. diamorphine subcutaneous infusion); O_2 if there is hypoxia; antibiotics if there is infection.
- Red cell transfusion for severe anaemia (sequestration or aplastic crisis) or as a 3–12-month programme of therapy for patients with frequently recurring crises or for 2–3 years following central nervous system crisis; or for patients in whom Doppler studies predict for stroke.

- Severe sickling or sequestration crisis (e.g. 'chest syndrome' and stroke) is treated acutely with exchange transfusion to reduce Hb S levels to <30%. Pregnant patients and those undergoing general anaesthesia may need transfusion to reduce Hb S levels to <30%.
- Oral hydroxyurea (20–40 mg/kg/day) reduces both the frequency and duration of sickle cell crises. Although its precise mode of action is not known, it increases Hb F production, decreases intracellular Hb S concentration by increasing mean corpuscular volume, lowers the neutrophil count and inhibits prothrombotic interactions between sickle cells and the endothelium.
- Stem cell transplantation in selected cases.
- Joint replacement surgery may be required for avascular necrosis (hips and shoulder).
- Iron chelation therapy for patients with iron overload caused by multiple transfusions.

Sickle cell trait

Sickle cell trait is a benign condition without anaemia and is usually asymptomatic. Occasionally haematuria or overt crisis occurs. Genetic counselling should be offered to carriers.

Other sickling disorders

Hb S may occur in combination with other genetic defects of haemoglobin (compound heterozygotes). Hb S/β-thalassaemia (Fig. 19c) clinically resembles Hb SS but the spleen usually remains enlarged and mean corpuscular volume is reduced. Hb SC disease varies in severity from mild to indistinguishable from sickle cell anaemia; thrombotic complications are particularly common.

Other structural haemoglobin abnormalities

Many other mutations of the α- or β-chain genes have been identified. Most that have a significant population frequency (e.g. Hb D) are not associated with clinical symptoms. However, some (e.g. Hb E) will cause significant disease in a homozygous state or if co-inherited with a β-thalassaemia allele.

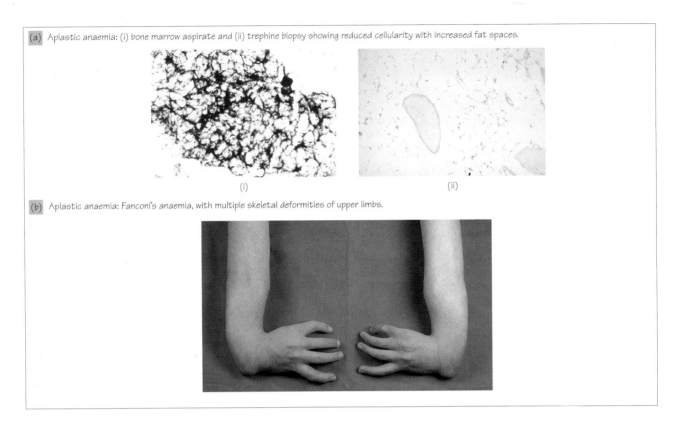

(a) Aplastic anaemia: (i) bone marrow aspirate and (ii) trephine biopsy showing reduced cellularity with increased fat spaces.

(i)　　　　　　(ii)

(b) Aplastic anaemia: Fanconi's anaemia, with multiple skeletal deformities of upper limbs.

Introduction

Bone marrow failure is the inability of the bone marrow to produce sufficient red cells, white cells and platelets resulting in pancytopenia (reduction in the blood of red cells, white cells and platelets). Causes are listed in Table 20.1. It occurs most commonly after the administration of chemotherapy and radiotherapy for the treatment of haemopoietic malignancies.

Clinical features

- Symptoms and signs of anaemia, infections and easy bruising or bleeding.
- Symptoms and signs as a result of the underlying cause, e.g. side effects of chemotherapy.

Laboratory findings

- Anaemia, leucopenia and thrombocytopenia of varying severity.
- Blood film typically shows no abnormal cells. It may show circulating red cell and white precursors (leucoerythroblastic) caused by bone marrow infiltration (see Chapter 42) or may show evidence of a primary haematological malignancy, e.g. leukaemia.
- Bone marrow aspirate and trephine biopsy are required to define cause (Fig. 20a).

Differential diagnosis

Pancytopenia can also result from accelerated destruction of cells (e.g. as a result of splenomegaly or autoimmune destruction) or pooling of cells (e.g. within an enlarged spleen).

Treatment

- Remove any known cause, e.g. drugs.
- Support care with appropriate blood components and antimicrobials (see Chapters 46, 47 and 49).
- Specific therapy is considered separately with the specific diseases.

Aplastic anaemia

This is a chronic pancytopenia associated with a hypoplastic bone marrow. There are reduced marrow stem cells, increased fat spaces (fat/haemopoiesis ratio >75:25%) and no abnormal cells present.

Aetiology and pathogenesis

The disease may be congenital or acquired (Table 20.2).
- Congenital aplastic anaemia may be inherited as an autosomal recessive (Fanconi type); rarely associated with dyskeratosis congenita (which may be either sex linked or autosomal recessive).

46 *Haematology at a Glance*, 3e. By A. Mehta and V. Hoffbrand. Published 2009 by Blackwell Publishing. ISBN 978-1-4051-7970-6.

Table 20.1 Bone marrow failure

Primary reduction in haemopoietic cells
Aplastic anaemia
Chemotherapy, radiotherapy

Replacement of marrow by malignant cells
Primary – leukaemia, myeloma, lymphoma
Secondary, e.g. carcinoma

Ineffective haemopoiesis
Myelodysplasia, megaloblastic anaemia

Infiltration by abnormal tissue
Myelofibrosis
Rarely, Gaucher's disease, amyloidosis, osteopetrosis

• Acquired aplastic anaemia has an identifiable cause (viral infection, radiation or drug exposure) in about 50% of cases. In the remainder, the cause is unknown but may involve an immune reaction against marrow stem cells.

Clinical features
• May occur at any age, in either sex, incidence of 2–5 cases per million population.
• Onset rapid (over a few days) or slow (over weeks or months).
• Symptoms and signs are caused by bone marrow failure (see above).
• Liver, spleen and lymph nodes are not enlarged.
• Fanconi's anaemia (Fig. 20b) usually presents in childhood. Associated findings may include skeletal and renal tract defects, microcephaly and altered skin pigmentation. In dyskeratosis congenita, there are skin, hair and nail changes.

Laboratory findings
• Anaemia is normocytic or mildly macrocytic with a low reticulocyte count.
• Leucopenia is usual with neutrophils below 1.5×10^9/L ($<0.2 \times 10^9$/L in severe cases).
• Thrombocytopenia ($<10 \times 10^9$/L in severe cases).

Table 20.2 Causes of aplastic anaemia

Congenital
Fanconi
Other, e.g. dyskeratosis congenita

Acquired
Idiopathic
Secondary
  Inevitable (cytotoxic drugs, radiation)
  Idiosyncratic
  Drugs, e.g. chloramphenicol, sulphonamides, gold, chlorpromazine, carbimazole
  Chemical agents/toxins, e.g. benzene
  Infection, e.g. viral hepatitis (non-A, non-B, non-C)
Associated with haematological malignancy, e.g. acute lymphoblastic leukaemia
Other, e.g. in association with paroxysmal nocturnal haemoglobinuria

• Bone marrow is hypoplastic with >75% fat spaces. Remaining haemopoietic cells are of normal appearance. Megakaryocytes are particularly reduced.
• In Fanconi's anaemia lymphocyte chromosomes show random breaks.

Specific therapy
• Immunosuppression, e.g. antilymphocyte globulin (ALG), horse or rabbit, given intravenously over several days, and cyclosporin (alone or with ALG) improve marrow function in 50–70% of severe cases. ALG is given with corticosteroids to prevent serum sickness
• Androgens (e.g. oxymetholone) may benefit Fanconi's anaemia and acquired aplastic anaemia.
• Stem cell transplantation offers a cure in severe cases. This requires an HLA matching sibling or unrelated matching volunteer to act as donor. Results are best (60–70% cure) in younger patients (<20 yr).
• Haemopoietic growth factors, granulocyte colony-stimulating factor, may raise the neutrophil count temporarily but has no long-term benefit on the underlying bone marrow defect.
• Blood product support (Chapter 46).

Red cell aplasia
Red cell aplasia is anaemia caused by selective reduction of red cell production by the bone marrow. There is absence or severe reduction of developing erythroblasts in the marrow and of reticulocytes in the peripheral blood, with no abnormality in other cell lines.

Clinical and laboratory features
A rare congenital form (Diamond–Blackfan anaemia, due to a defect in ribosome function) is frequently associated with other somatic malformations. Acquired red cell aplasia may occur as a result of drugs (e.g. azathioprine, isoniazid), in association with autoimmune diseases (e.g. systemic lupus erythematosus), haematological malignancy (e.g. chronic lymphocytic leukaemia) or with a thymoma (see Chapter 42).

Transient red cell aplasia occurs following infection with B19 parvovirus and can lead to a profound but temporary reduction of red cell production with severe anaemia in patients with a haemolytic disorder (e.g. 'aplastic crisis' in hereditary spherocytosis or sickle cell anaemia).

Treatment
Treatment of the underlying disorder (e.g. removal of a thymoma) is required. Red cell transfusion and iron chelation therapy may be required. Immunosuppressive therapy (e.g. prednisolone, cyclosporin, ALG or rituximab) is useful in selected patients with either congenital or acquired red cell aplasia.

Congenital dyserythropoietic anaemias
Congenital dyserythropoietic anaemias are a rare group of recessively inherited conditions in which chronic anaemia results from abnormal maturation of erythroid cells in the marrow. Red cell precursors usually show marked morphological abnormalities, e.g. bi- and trinucleated normoblasts.

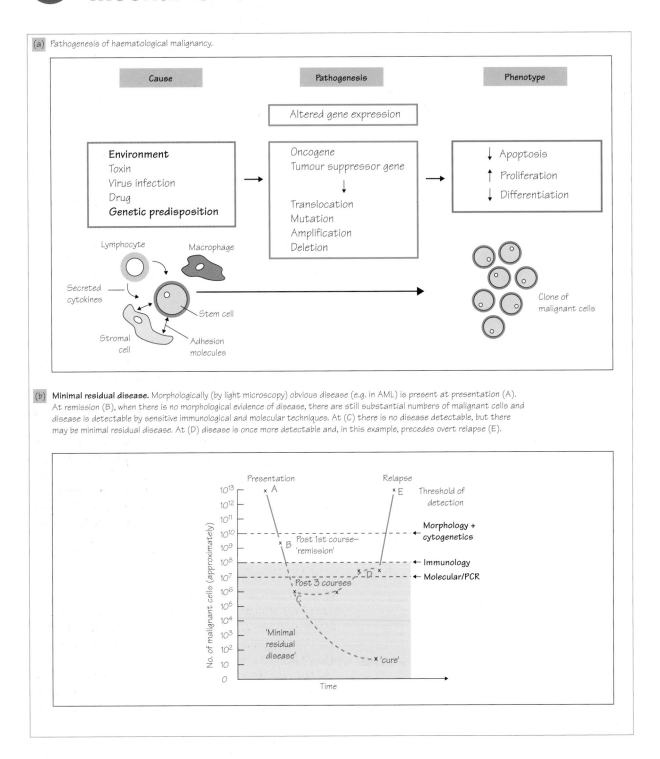

(a) Pathogenesis of haematological malignancy.

(b) **Minimal residual disease.** Morphologically (by light microscopy) obvious disease (e.g. in AML) is present at presentation (A). At remission (B), when there is no morphological evidence of disease, there are still substantial numbers of malignant cells and disease is detectable by sensitive immunological and molecular techniques. At (C) there is no disease detectable, but there may be minimal residual disease. At (D) disease is once more detectable and, in this example, precedes overt relapse (E).

Neoplasia

Haematological malignancies (Table 21.1) are thought to arise from a single cell in the bone marrow, thymus or peripheral lymphoid system which has undergone one or more genetic change (somatic mutation) leading to malignant *transformation*. Successive mitotic divisions give rise to a clone of cells derived from the parent cell. Further mutations may give rise to sub-clones (clonal evolution). Transformed cells proliferate excessively and/or are resistant to apoptosis. They are often 'frozen' at a particular stage of differentiation. 'Acute' malignancies are those that appear and progress over a short timescale (days or weeks) and the tumour cells are usually morphologically immature ('blasts'). They require immediate treatment. Chronic malignancies appear and progress over a longer timescale (months

Table 21.1 Classification of haematological malignancies

	Acute	Chronic
Lymphoid	ALL and subtypes	Chronic lymphocytic leukaemia
		NHL
		HL
		Multiple myeloma and variants
Myeloid	AML and subtypes	CML
		MDS
		Myeloproliferative disorders

ALL, acute lymphoblastic leukaemia; NHL, non-Hodgkin lymphoma; HL, Hodgkin lymphoma; AML, acute myeloid leukaemia; CML, chronic myeloid leukaemia; MDS, myelodysplasia.

or years), and the tumour cells are often difficult to distinguish morphologically from normal cells; they do not always require immediate treatment.

Causes of neoplasia

Neoplasia is caused by a complex interaction between genetic and environmental mechanisms (Fig. 21a).

• Genetic predisposition. Certain inherited conditions, e.g. Down's syndrome, trisomy 21 and conditions associated with defective DNA repair, e.g. Fanconi's anaemia or immune suppression e.g. ataxia telangiectasia.

• Viral infection. Human T-cell leukaemia virus (HTLV-1) incorporates into T-lymphoid cell genome and underlies adult T-cell leukaemia lymphoma (see Chapter 33). Other viruses predispose to malignancy by immune suppression (e.g. HIV). Epidemiological evidence implicates Epstein–Barr virus in Burkitt's lymphoma and less strongly with Hodgkin's disease. *Helicobacter pylori* infection of the stomach predisposes to gastric lymphoma.

• Ionizing radiation causes DNA mutation and increases the risk of haematological neoplasia.

• Toxins/chemicals, e.g. benzene and organochemicals may predispose to leukaemia and myelodysplasia (MDS).

• Drugs. Alkylating agents (e.g. melphalan, mustine) and other forms of chemotherapy predispose to MDS or acute myeloid leukaemia.

Mechanism of malignant transformation

Altered expression of two types of gene underlies multistep pathogenesis of haematological malignancy.

Oncogenes

Oncogenes, whose protein products cause malignant transformation, are derived from normal cellular genes (proto-oncogenes). These codes for proteins usually involved in one or other stage in cell signal transduction, gene transcription, cell cycle, cell survival/apoptosis or differentiation. Activation of proto-oncogenes to become oncogenes may occur by **amplification**, **point mutation** or **translocation** from

one chromosomal location to another. Translocation is most frequent in haematological malignancies and may lead to a quantitative change in expression (e.g. MYC translocation to the immunoglobulin heavy chain locus in lymphoid neoplasia, t(8;14) or of the BCL-2 gene (which inhibits apoptosis) in follicular lymphoma). Translocation may also lead to a qualitative change by joining all or part of the oncogene to another gene to form a fusion gene (e.g. ABL translocation from chromosome 9 to the breakpoint cluster region (BCR) on chromosome 22 to form BCR-ABL in CML, t(9;22)).

Anti-oncogenes (tumour suppressor genes)

These are genes encoding proteins which have a critical role in suppressing cell growth. Chromosome deletion may obliterate tumour suppressor genes on one allele; deletion or mutation of the remaining allele may allow uncontrolled cell growth.

Micro-RNAs

Micro-RNAs are synthesised from genes distributed throughout the genome. They affect transcription and are deleted in some deletions, e.g. 13q in chronic lymphocytic leukaemia.

Evidence of clonality

A population of cells is considered clonal (derived from a single cell by mitotic division) if they have some or all the following features.

• The same acquired chromosome abnormality, e.g. Ph chromosome (see Fig. 21a) or point mutation within an individual gene.

• Clonal rearrangement of an immunoglobulin or T-cell receptor gene in lymphoid neoplasia.

• Restriction in a B-lymphoid neoplasm to expression of only λ or only κ light chains, but not both as in polyclonal B cells.

• Restriction fragment length polymorphism in which the size of a restriction fragment of DNA on the X chromosome is analysed. In females, two fragments derived from the two X chromosomes will be found in polyclonal populations, both fragments being hypomethylated and transcriptionally active. In tumours only one size of fragment is hypomethylated as only one X chromosome is active.

Minimal residual disease

At the time of diagnosis of a haematological neoplasm, the patient will have approximately 10^{13}–10^{14} malignant cells. Even if treatment results in 1000-fold reduction of tumour cells, there remain 10^{10} cells, which may be below the microscopic level of detection. Using immunological or molecular techniques, minimal residual disease (MRD) may be detected in blood or marrow of patients who clinically and by conventional light microscopy are in complete remission (Fig. 21b).

The techniques to detect MRD include:

• immunological (e.g. flow cytometry) particularly if residual malignant cells carry a distinctively abnormal phenotype (pattern of antigen expression);

• chromosomal analysis and fluorescence in situ hybridization (see Chapter 7) and

• molecular using the polymerase chain reaction, which is the most sensitive (will detect one malignant cell in up to 10^6 normal cells).

Acute leukaemia I: classification and diagnosis

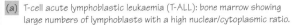

(a) T-cell acute lymphoblastic leukaemia (T-ALL): bone marrow showing large numbers of lymphoblasts with a high nuclear/cytoplasmic ratio.

(b) B-cell ALL: bone marrow showing large blasts with characteristic vacuoles and blue cytoplasm.

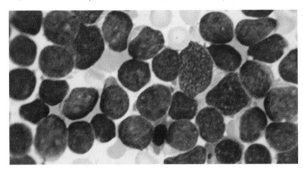

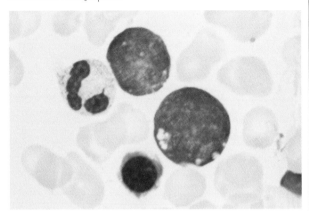

(c) Precursor B-ALL: cerebrospinal fluid cytocentrifuge specimen showing lymphoblasts.

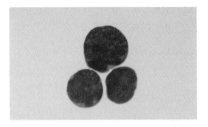

Acute leukaemia is a malignant disorder in which haemopoietic blast cells constitute >20% of bone marrow cells. The primitive cells usually also accumulate in the blood, infiltrate other tissues and cause bone marrow failure.

Classification

There are two main groups: acute lymphoblastic (ALL) and acute myeloid (myeloblastic) leukaemia (AML). Rare cases are undifferentiated or mixed. Subclassification of ALL or AML depends on morphological, immunological, cytochemical and cytogenetic criteria (Tables 22.1–22.3).

Aetiology and pathogenesis

The malignant cells typically show a chromosome translocation or other DNA mutation affecting oncogenes (see Chapter 21). AML may follow previous myeloproliferative or myelodysplastic diseases. In childhood B lineage (precursor B), ALL there is evidence from identical twin studies that the first event, a chromosomal translocation, may occur *in utero* and a subsequent second event (e.g. infection) precipitates the onset of ALL.

Incidence

Approximately 1000 new cases (20–25 per million population) each of AML and ALL per year in the UK. ALL is the most common malignancy in childhood (peak age of 4 yr) but also occurs in adults. AML occurs at all ages but is rarer than ALL in childhood, being most common in the elderly.

Clinical features

• Short (<3 mo) history of symptoms due to bone marrow failure (e.g. of anaemia, abnormal bruising/bleeding or infection). Disseminated intravascular coagulation (DIC) with bleeding is particularly common in promyelocytic AML t(15;17).
• Increased cellular catabolism may cause sweating, fever and general malaise.
• Lymphadenopathy and hepatosplenomegaly are frequent, especially in ALL.
• Tissue infiltration, e.g. of meninges, testes (more common in ALL), skin, bones, gums with hypertrophy (AML with monocytic differentiation) may cause clinical symptoms or signs.

Laboratory features

• Anaemia, thrombocytopenia and often neutropenia.
• Leucocytosis caused by blast cells in the blood usually occurs. Leucopenia is less frequent.
• The bone marrow shows infiltration by blast cells (>20% and often 80–90% of marrow cells).
• Coagulation may be abnormal and DIC can occur, especially with acute promyelocytic leukaemia.
• Serum uric acid, lactate dehydrogenase (LD) may be raised.
• Morphological analysis (ALL Figs 22a–c; AML Figs 22d–j) usually reveals cytoplasmic granules or Auer rods (condensations of granules) in AML. Cytochemical stains are helpful – AML blasts have granules positive by Sudan black, myeloperoxidase and chloroacetate esterase, while monoblasts are positive for non-specific and butyrate esterase. B-lineage lymphoblasts

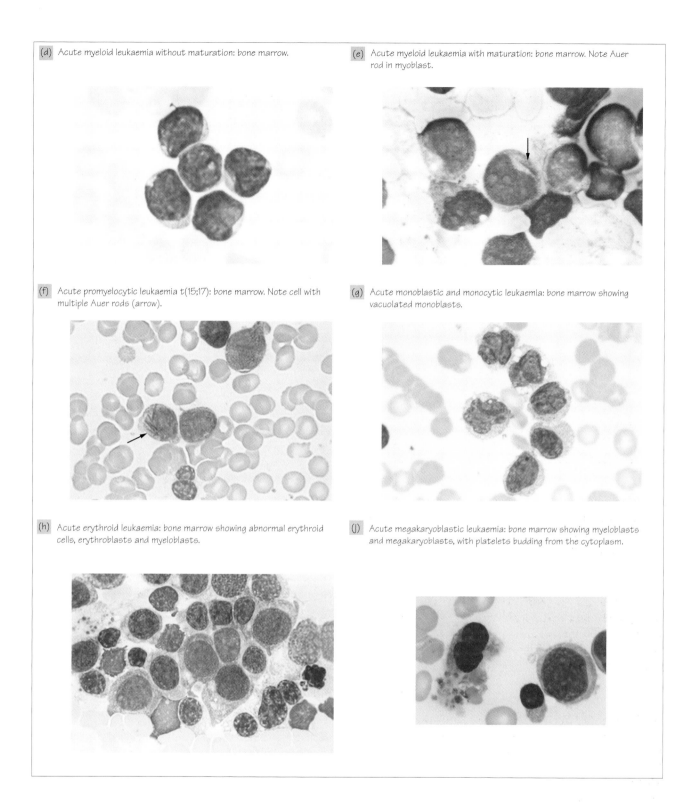

(d) Acute myeloid leukaemia without maturation: bone marrow.

(e) Acute myeloid leukaemia with maturation: bone marrow. Note Auer rod in myoblast.

(f) Acute promyelocytic leukaemia t(15;17): bone marrow. Note cell with multiple Auer rods (arrow).

(g) Acute monoblastic and monocytic leukaemia: bone marrow showing vacuolated monoblasts.

(h) Acute erythroid leukaemia: bone marrow showing abnormal erythroid cells, erythroblasts and myeloblasts.

(j) Acute megakaryoblastic leukaemia: bone marrow showing myeloblasts and megakaryoblasts, with platelets budding from the cytoplasm.

show blocks of positive material with periodic acid–Schiff (PAS) stain, and in T-lineage ALL with acid phosphatase.

• Immunophenotype analysis involves the use of antibodies and fluorescence-activated cell sorting to identify cell antigens (many termed clusters of differentiation or CD, see Appendix III) which correlate with lineage and maturity (Table 22.2). Other antigens, e.g. TdT, and cytoplasmic immunoglobulin may be also be detected.

• Cytogenetic and DNA microarray analysis gives diagnostic and prognostic information (Tables 22.3 and 22.4).

• Cases with normal cytogenetics may be subclassified into whether or not they show mutations of genes NPM1, FLT3, CEBPA and other genes which have prognostic significance (Table 22.3).

Table 22.1 WHO (2008) classification of acute leukaemia (simplified)

AMLs
  AML with recurrent cytogenetic abnormalities
    AML with t(8,21) (*AML1/ETO*)
    Acute promyelocytic leukaemia with t(15,17) (*PML/RARA*)
    AML with abnormal bone marrow eosinophils inv 16 (*CBFbeta/MYH11*)
    AML with 11q23 (*MLL*) abnormalities
    AML with other abnormalities, e.g. t(6;9), inv (3), t(1;22)
  AML with myelodysplasia-related features
  Therapy-related myeloid neoplasms
  AML with mutated NPMI or CEBPA
  AML not otherwise categorized
    AML with minimal differentiation
    AML without maturation
    AML with maturation
    Acute myelomonocytic leukaemia
    Acute monoblastic and monocytic leukaemia
    Acute erythroid, erythroid/myeloid, megakaryoblastic/basophilic leukaemia
  Acute panmyelosis with myelofibrosis
  Acute leukaemia of ambiguous lineage (undifferentiated or biphenotypic)
  Myeloid sarcoma

ALL
  Precursor B-cell lymphoblastic leukaemia/lymphoma
    Unspecified
    With recurrent cytogenetic/molecular genetic abnormalities, e.g. t(9;22), t(v;11q23), t(12;21), hyperdiploidy, hypodiploidy, t(1;19)
  Precursor T-cell lymphoblastic leukaemia/lymphoma

ALL, acute lymphoblastic leukaemia; AML, acute myeloid leukaemia
NB: The WHO classification also includes myeloid proliferations related to Down's syndrome which may be transient

Table 22.2 Immunophenotypes of acute leukaemia

Disease	Immunophenotype
AML	CD33, CD13
	Monocytic cells: CD14, CD61
	Megakaryoblasts: CD41, CD61
	Erythroid: glycophorin, transferrin receptor (CD71)
ALL	
B-cell precursor	CD19, TdT
(More mature)	CD10, CD19, CD20, cyt CD22, TdT, cyIg/sMIg
T-cell precursor	CD7, cyt CD3, TdT

CD34 is a marker of haemopoietic stem cells and may be positive in both AML and ALL
ALL, acute lymphoblastic leukaemia; AML, acute myeloid leukaemia; CyIg, cytoplasmic immunoglobin; sMIg, surface membrane immunoglobulin; TdT, terminal deoxynucleotidyl transferase

Table 22.3 Prognostic indicators in acute myeloid leukaemia

Good risk
  Cytogenetic changes: (8,21), t(15,17), inversion 16
  Molecular changes: mutations in nucleophosmin gene (NPM)

Poor risk
  Cytogenetic changes: Monosomy 5, monosomy 7 Complex karyotypes, 11q 23 abnormalities
  Molecular changes: Mutations of Flt-3 gene

Standard risk
  All other cases. These cases may be further subdivided into prognostic groups using DNA microarray techniques.

MDR, multi-drug resistance

Table 22.4 Prognostic factors in acute lymphoblastic leukaemia

	Good	Bad
Sex	Female	Male
Age	2–9 yr	Adult
White cell count	Low ($<10 \times 10^9$/L)	High ($>50 \times 10^9$/L)
Chromosomes	Hyperdiploid	t(9;22), t(4;11)
Extramedullary disease	Absent	Present
Speed of remission	4 weeks	>4 weeks
Clearance of peripheral blood blasts	1 week	>1 week
Loss of minimal residual disease in bone marrow	1–3 mo	3–6 mo or more

Acute leukaemia II: treatment and prognosis

Treatment

The first phase of therapy (remission induction) is with high-dose intensive combination chemotherapy to reduce or eradicate leukaemic cells from the bone marrow and reestablish normal haemopoiesis. Further therapy is post-induction chemotherapy; this may be intensive ('intensification' or 'consolidation' chemotherapy) or less intensive (maintenance chemotherapy). Each course of intensive treatment typically requires 4–6 weeks in hospital. Complications of chemotherapy and supportive care are considered in Chapter 49; blood component therapy is considered in Chapter 46.

Acute myeloid leukaemia

Remission induction regimes usually comprise an anthracycline (e.g. daunorubicin), cytosine arabinoside (ara-C) and in some protocols, etoposide. Fludarabine combined with high dose of ara-C and G-CSF (FLAG) may also be used for induction. All-*trans* retinoic acid (ATRA) is given concurrently in acute promyelocytic leukaemia (APML) to induce differentiation; arsenic trioxide is also active in this condition. More than 80% of patients under the age of 60 years achieve remission, defined as a normal full blood count and <5% blasts in bone marrow, with one course and >85% with two courses. Older patients and those with preceding myelodysplasia or acute myeloid (myeloblastic) leukaemia (AML) secondary to another disease (e.g. myeloproliferative disorder, MPD) have lower remission rates. Three further courses are usually given as post-induction therapy to younger (<60 yr) patients, and other agents used include mitoxantrone, M-AMSA, idarubicin and high-dose ara-C. Tumour lysis syndrome may occur (see p. 107) and APML patients are at high risk of developing DIC (see p. 84). Anti-CD33 monoclonal antibody combined with a toxin is undergoing trials. Some older patients may be considered medically unfit for intensive chemotherapy and may be treated with supportive care alone or with single agent palliative chemotherapy.

Acute lymphoblastic leukaemia

Remission induction regimes comprise vincristine, prednisolone and L-asparaginase often with daunorubicin, cyclophosphamide.

Post-remission therapy is with two or three 'intensification' blocks with additional drugs. Patients then receive maintenance chemotherapy for a further 2–3 years with daily mercaptopurine, weekly methotrexate and monthly vincristine and dexamethasone. Treatment protocols may be modified according to whether minimal residual disease can be detected at various time points in therapy.

Central nervous system involvement is common in acute lymphoblastic leukaemia (ALL) in children and adults, and normal practice is to give multiple intrathecal injections and courses of high-dose systemic chemotherapy with methotrexate or ara-C, or cranial radiotherapy to prevent or treat this complication.

Stem cell transplantation (see Chapter 48)

Allogeneic stem cell transplantation (SCT) is recommended for selected adult patients (<60 yr) in first remission of AML and for adults with ALL (>20 yr and <50 yr) who have a histocompatible sibling. Transplants using matched unrelated volunteer donors are being increasingly performed. However, good prognosis AML (Table 22.3) and ALL (Table 22.4) cases are not given SCT in first remission.

Prognosis

Childhood acute lymphoblastic leukaemia

Overall 80% of children with ALL are cured, the best responses being in girls, aged 2–12 years with low presenting white cell count ($<10 \times 10^9$/L) and favourable cytogenetics (Table 22.4).

Acute myeloid leukaemia and adult acute lymphoblastic leukaemia

Approximately 30–40% of patients less than 60 years old are cured. This varies widely according to age and prognostic features. Results are improving in the 60–70-year-old group, but over 70 years less than 10% are cured.

Long-term complications of treatment

Increasing cure rates mean that these are relevant for all children and most adults. They are considered in Chapter 50.

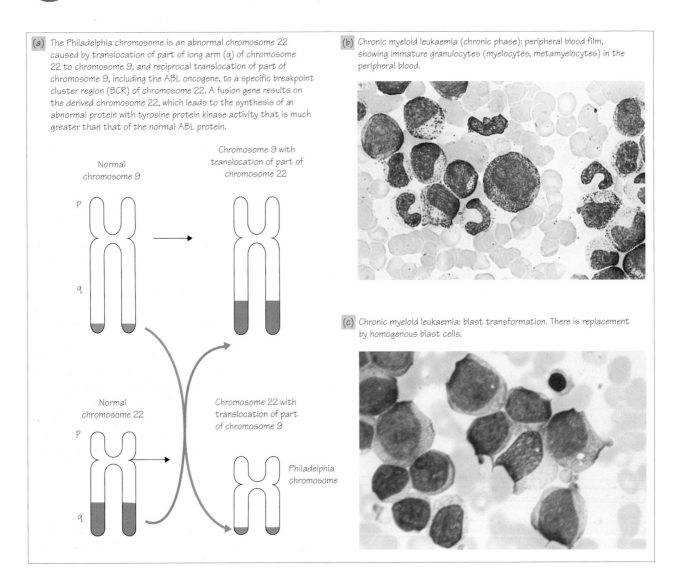

(a) The Philadelphia chromosome is an abnormal chromosome 22 caused by translocation of part of long arm (q) of chromosome 22 to chromosome 9, and reciprocal translocation of part of chromosome 9, including the ABL oncogene, to a specific breakpoint cluster region (BCR) of chromosome 22. A fusion gene results on the derived chromosome 22, which leads to the synthesis of an abnormal protein with tyrosine protein kinase activity that is much greater than that of the normal ABL protein.

Normal chromosome 9

Chromosome 9 with translocation of part of chromosome 22

Normal chromosome 22

Chromosome 22 with translocation of part of chromosome 9

Philadelphia chromosome

(b) Chronic myeloid leukaemia (chronic phase): peripheral blood film, showing immature granulocytes (myelocytes, metamyelocytes) in the peripheral blood.

(c) Chronic myeloid leukaemia: blast transformation. There is replacement by homogenous blast cells.

This is a clonal myeloproliferative disorder characterized by an increase in neutrophils and their precursors in the peripheral blood with increased cellularity of the marrow as a result of an excess of granulocyte precursors. The leukaemic cells of >95% of patients have a reciprocal translocation between the long arms of chromosomes 9 and 22, t(9;22). The derived chromosome 22 is termed the Philadelphia (Ph) chromosome (Fig. 24a). The disease may transform from a relatively stable chronic phase to an acute leukaemia phase (blast transformation).

Aetiology and pathophysiology

Aetiology is unknown. Exposure to ionizing radiation is a risk factor. The ABL oncogene is translocated from chromosome 9 into the breakpoint cluster region (BCR) on chromosome 22 to form the *BCR-ABL* fusion gene (see Fig. 24a) This fusion gene encodes a 210-kDa protein with greatly increased tyrosine kinase activity compared to the normal ABL product. The disease is of stem cell origin as the Ph chromosome is present in erythroid, granulocytic, megakaryocytic and T-lymphoid precursors. Rare cases show variant translocations or are Ph-negative but show the *BCR-ABL* fusion gene. The Ph chromosome abnormality may also occur in acute lymphoblastic leukaemia (ALL; see Chapter 22).

Clinical features

- Occur at all ages (peak age of 25–45 yr, male/female ratio equal, incidence of 5–10 cases per million population).
- Patients usually present in the chronic phase.
- Presenting symptoms include weight loss, night sweats, itching, left hypochondrial pain, gout.
- Priapism, visual disturbance and headaches caused by hyperviscosity (WBC >250 × 10^9/L) are less frequent.
- Splenomegaly, often massive, occurs in over 90% of cases.
- Some cases are discovered on routine blood test.

Laboratory findings

- Raised white cell count (often 50×10^9/L or more), mainly neutrophils and myelocytes (Fig. 24b).
- Basophils may be prominent.
- Platelet count may be raised, normal or low and anaemia may be present.
- Raised serum uric acid.
- Bone marrow is hypercellular with a raised myeloid/erythroid ratio (see Chapter 1).
- Cytogenetic analysis of bone marrow cells shows the Ph chromosome in >95% of metaphases. The *BCR-ABL* fusion gene is detectable by FISH and its RNA product by PCR (see Chapter 7).

Course and progress

Patients are typically well during the 'chronic phase'. Main cause of death is transformation into acute leukaemia (Fig. 24c) (80% AML, 20% ALL, with a proportion showing a mixed blast cell population), which may occur at any stage, even at presentation. Median survival is currently more than 6 years. Staging to predict prognosis has been attempted using age, spleen size, blood blast cell and platelet counts. There may be an accelerated phase of variable duration in which anaemia, thrombocytopenia, splenic enlargement and marrow fibrosis occur. Transformation is usually accompanied by additional morphological and new chromosome abnormalities.

Treatment

Chronic phase

Imatinib (Glivec)

- This is a specific inhibitor of the tyrosine kinase encoded by BCR-ABL. It controls the blood count and causes the marrow to become Ph negative in a high proportion of cases; the patients with the best responses become negative for the *BCR-ABL* fusion gene when tested by PCR and >95% will still be alive 6 years after diagnosis. The duration of the chronic phase is prolonged in nearly all patients and rate of acute transformation is greatly reduced. Side effects include nausea, skin rashes and muscle pains. Imatinib in combination with other drugs is also valuable in therapy of Ph + ALL and blast transformation of CML.
- Newer tyrosine kinase inhibitors include nilotinib and dasatinib. They may be more active than imatinib in patients with acute transformation. They also have activity in patients with CML who are resistant to imatinib.
- Imatinib and the newer drugs have made a major impact on the prognosis for patients with CML and have changed the paradigm for leukaemia sufferers worldwide. Many leukaemias – and other types of cancer – have become chronic diseases, controllable with long-term pharmacological approaches. Imatinib is one of the most expensive prescription medications available worldwide, and its development and successful adoption have caused healthcare systems re-appraise procedures for reimbursement of the costs of medication.
- Hydroxycarbamide (hydroxyurea) will control the raised white cell count and may be used initially before starting imatinib.
- α-Interferon (IFN) may also control the white cell count and may delay onset of acute transformation, prolonging overall survival by 1–2 years. The best responders to IFN become Ph negative, but usually remain BCR-ABL positive, and have the best prognosis. Combination therapies, e.g. IFN − imatinib, IFN + cytosine arabinoside, are more effective than IFN alone.
- Allopurinol to prevent hyperuricaemia.
- Allogeneic stem cell transplantation (SCT) before the age of 50 from an HLA-matching sibling offers a 70% chance of cure in chronic phase, but 30% or less once acceleration has occurred. The advent of imatinib makes the risks of SCT less acceptable and SCT is reserved for the minority of patients who do not respond to imatinib or are already in accelerated or acute phase presentation. HLA-matched unrelated donor SCT is less successful in curing the disease because of higher morbidity and mortality. Transfusion of donor lymphocytes may be valuable in eliminating BCR-ABL-positive cells in case of relapse post-SCT.

Acute phase

This is now much rarer with the widespread use of imatinib.

Therapy as for acute leukaemia, AML or ALL with addition of imatinib may be given, SCT may also be tried but the prognosis is poor.

Rare variants of CML include chronic neutrophilic eosinophilic and basophilic leukaemias. These are BCR-ABL negative and do not respond to imatinib.

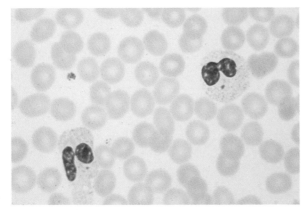

(a) Myelodysplasia: peripheral blood film showing hypogranular neutrophils with bilobed nuclei (pseudo-Pelger cells).

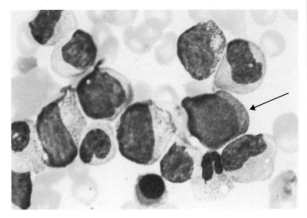

(b) Myelodysplasia: bone marrow aspirate showing a granular blast with blue cytoplasm (arrow) and hypogranular maturing myeloid cells.

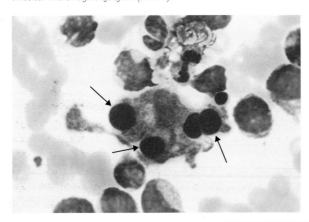

(c) Myelodysplasia: bone marrow aspirate showing mononuclear and binuclear micromegakaryocytes (arrows).

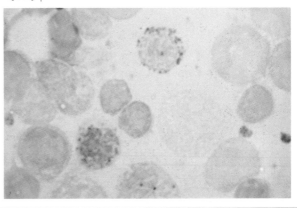

(d) Iron (Perls') stain of bone marrow aspirate showing iron granules in a perinuclear distribution (ringed sideroblasts) from a patients with myelodysplasia.

This is a clonal haemopoietic stem cell disorder characterized by peripheral blood cytopenias usually affecting more than one lineage usually in association with a hypercellular marrow, indicating ineffective haemopoiesis.

Aetiology and pathogenesis

Myelodysplasia (MDS) may be primary (*de novo*) or a consequence of previous chemotherapy/radiotherapy (secondary). Various chromosome and oncogene abnormalities occur, e.g. complete or partial deletions of chromosomes 5 or 7, point mutations in RAS oncogenes. The disease is divided into seven subgroups (Table 25.1). It may transform to acute myeloid leukaemia (AML) (>20% blasts in the marrow).

Clinical features

- Most frequent in the elderly, but young adults or even children may be affected.
- Bone marrow failure (see Chapter 20) with anaemia and/or leucopenia and/or thrombocytopenia.

- The 5q-syndrome is a subgroup, occurring particularly in elderly females with a high platelet count, macrocytosis and good prognosis.

Laboratory findings

- Anaemia is usually macrocytic.
- Neutropenia is frequent and neutrophils may be hypogranular with pseudo-Pelger forms (Fig. 25a).
- Bone marrow is usually hypercellular but may be hypocellular and/or fibrotic.
- Characteristic morphological changes are seen in all three lineages (Figs. 25a–25c).

Differential diagnosis

This is very broad, particularly when only one lineage is involved in an elderly person. Thus, other causes of anaemia must be excluded. Thrombocytopenia or leucopenia may be caused by drugs, immune destruction or hypersplenism. The hallmark of MDS is involvement of more than one – typically all three –

Table 25.1 Classification of the myelodysplastic and myelodysplastic/myeloproliferative syndromes

Myelodysplastic syndromes
  Refractory cytopenias with uni-lineage dysplasia
    Refractory anaemia
    Refractory neutropenia
    Refractory thrombocytopenia
  Refractory anaemia with ring sideroblasts
  Refractory cytopenia with multi-lineage dysplasia
  Refractory anaemia with excess blasts
  Myelodysplastic syndromes associated with isolated del (5q)
  Myelodysplastic syndromes, unclassifiable
  Myelodysplastic syndromes in children

Myelodysplastic/Myeloproliferative neoplasms
  Chronic myelomonocytic leukaemia
  Atypical chronic myeloid leukaemia, BCR-ABL negative
  Juvenile myelomonocytic leukaemia
  Refractory anaemia with ring sideroblasts (RARS) associated with marked thrombocytosis
  Myelodysplastic/myeloproliferative neoplasms unclassifiable

lineage(s). Nevertheless, distinction between MDS, myelofibrosis and aplasia may be difficult in patients with pancytopenia. The finding of a cytogenetic abnormality greatly strengthens what may otherwise be a subjective morphological diagnosis.

Course and prognosis

This depends on the type of MDS (see Table 25.1). The degree of cytopenia influences the incidence of complications and treatment, while the percentage of blast cells is predictive of the risk of developing acute leukaemia. The presence of complex cytogenetic changes is also associated with a poor prognosis. Scoring systems have been devised whereby the degree of cytopenia, proportion of blasts and nature of cytogenetic changes are used to estimate prognosis. These scoring systems are helpful in planning treatment as they help patients, their carers and physicians in making complex decisions whereby the risks of treatment must be balanced against the risk of disease progression. Death may be caused by infection, haemorrhage, iron overload from multiple transfusions or from transformation into AML.

Treatment

- Support care with red cell or platelet transfusions and antimicrobials may be required.
- Iron chelation therapy may be needed for multiply transfused iron loaded patients with an otherwise good prognosis.
- Granulocyte colony-stimulating factor may be used temporarily to increase neutrophil production; erythropoietin produces a rise in haemoglobin in about 5–15% of patients with refractory anaemia.
- Chemotherapy with low-dose ara-C, etoposide, hydroxycarbamide or 6-mercaptopurine is used to control excess blast proliferation in patients unsuitable for high-dose chemotherapy. Newer agents include azacytidine and the thalidomide derivative lenalidomide, which is particularly active in patients with 5q abnormalities.
- Younger patients with refractory anaemia with excess blasts (RAEB) may be treated as AML. Complete remissions are less frequent than in *de novo* AML.
- Allogeneic stem cell transplantation (sibling or matched unrelated donor) may cure younger patients.

Myelodysplastic/myeloproliferative diseases

These have many of the laboratory findings of myelodysplasia with a hypercellular marrow and dysplastic features in the different cell lineages. In chronic myelomonocytic leukaemia, there are $>1.0 \times 10^9$/L monocytes in the peripheral blood, the spleen may be enlarged and marrow blasts are up to 10%. Juvenile myelomonocyte leukaemia is associated with lymphadenopathy and eczematous rash.

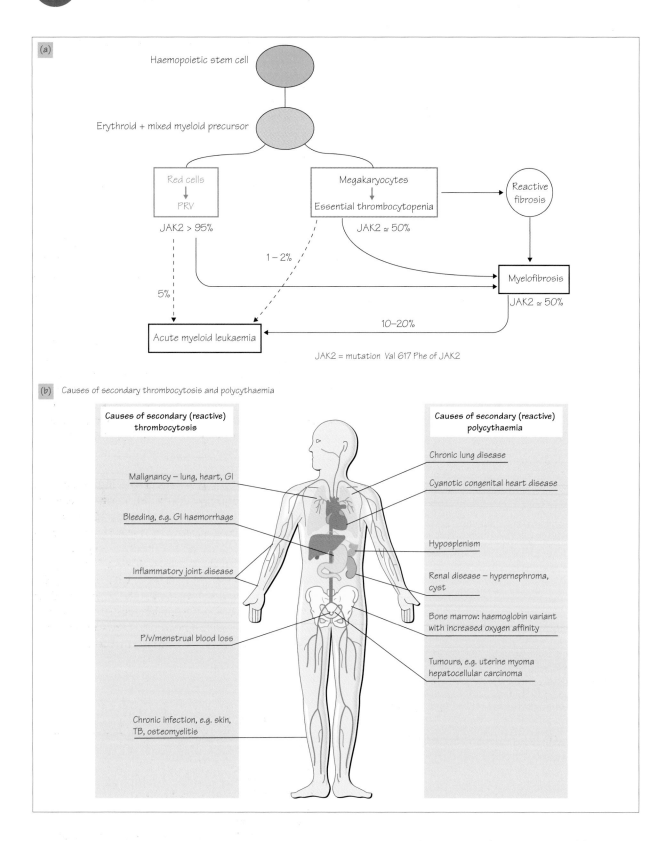

(a)

Haemopoietic stem cell

Erythroid + mixed myeloid precursor

Red cells
↓
PRV

JAK2 > 95%

Megakaryocytes

Essential thrombocytopenia

JAK2 ≃ 50%

Reactive fibrosis

1 – 2%

Myelofibrosis

JAK2 ≃ 50%

5%

10–20%

Acute myeloid leukaemia

JAK2 = mutation Val 617 Phe of JAK2

(b)   Causes of secondary thrombocytosis and polycythaemia

Causes of secondary (reactive) thrombocytosis

Malignancy – lung, heart, GI

Bleeding, e.g. GI haemorrhage

Inflammatory joint disease

P/v/menstrual blood loss

Chronic infection, e.g. skin, TB, osteomyelitis

Causes of secondary (reactive) polycythaemia

Chronic lung disease

Cyanotic congenital heart disease

Hyposplenism

Renal disease – hypernephroma, cyst

Bone marrow: haemoglobin variant with increased oxygen affinity

Tumours, e.g. uterine myoma hepatocellular carcinoma

Myeloproliferative disorders (MPD) are chronic diseases caused by clonal proliferation of bone marrow stem cells leading to excess production of one or more haemopoietic lineage. The clinical syndromes include polycythaemia rubra vera (PRV) (red cells), essential thrombocythaemia (ET) (platelets) and myelofibrosis in which there is a reactive fibrosis of the marrow and extramedullary haemopoiesis in the liver and spleen. Intermediate forms may occur and the diseases may all transform into acute myeloid leukaemia. A mutation (Val617Phe) of the Janus kinase 2 (JAK 2) is present in nearly 100% of cases of PRV and about 50% of cases of ET or myelofibrosis. It is usually heterozygous, but in 5–10% of positive cases, homozygous and these tend to be clinically more severe. Chronic myeloid leukaemia was formerly classified as an MPD but is now known to be due to a different mutation (BCR-ABL, see Chapter 24).

Differential diagnosis

Increased levels of red cells, white cells and platelets can occur in a range of physiolological and reactive conditions. Reactive causes of increased levels of white cells are considered in Chapter 9; reactive causes of increased levels of red cells, platelets and increased bone marrow fibrosis are listed in Tables 26.1–26.3 and illustrated in Figure 26 b. Careful clinical assessment is required to distinguish these reactive (secondary) conditions from primary myeloproliferative disorders in which there is an intrinsic disorder within the marrow stem cells. The general underlying mechanism is that an external stimulus leads to increased elaboration of erythropoietin and/or thrombopoietin (see Chapter 1). This leads to increased production of red cells and/or platelets by the bone marrow. This response may be physiological and appropriate (e.g. an increased Hb level in response to tissue hypoxia; or an increased platelet count in response to haemorrhage) or it may be pathological (e.g. increased red cell and/or platelet counts in response to ectopic production of hormones by tumours). The presence of a mutation within the JAK 2 locus or of a cytogenetic abnormality confirms that the patient is suffering from a primary myeloproliferative disorder.

Polycythaemia

Polycythaemia (erythrocytosis) is defined as an increase in red cell count or haemoglobin concentration above normal (Appendix II). True polycythaemia exists when the red cell mass (RCM), measured by dilution of isotopically labelled red cells, is increased above normal. Spurious (pseudo or stress) polycythaemia exists when an elevated haemoglobin concentration is caused by a reduction in plasma volume (see Table 26.1).

Thrombocytosis

Thrombocytosis is defined as an elevation of the blood platelet count above the normal range. Patients with polycythaemia or thrombocytosis are at an increased risk of thrombosis regardless of whether the underlying cause is reactive or a myeloproliferative disorder. Treatment of reactive polycythaemia, thrombocytosis and increased marrow fibrosis is usually directed at the underlying cause. Patients with reactive polycythaemia may require venesection but this should be done cautiously so that tissue oxygen requirements are not compromised. Patients with reactive thrombocytosis may require treatment with anti-platelet agents, e.g. aspirin, to reduce the risk of thrombosis.

Table 26.2 Causes of an elevated platelet count

Primary
Essential thrombocythaemia
As part of another myeloproliferative disorder, e.g. PRV, CML, myelofibrosis

Reactive
Iron deficiency
Haemorrhage
Severe haemolysis
Trauma, postoperatively
Infection, inflammation
Malignancy
Hyposplenism

CML, chronic myeloid leukaemia; PRV, polycythaemia rubra vera.

Table 26.1 Causes of polycythaemia

True polycythaemia
　Primary
　　PRV
　Secondary
　Erythropoietin appropriately increased
　　High altitude
　　Cyanotic congenital heart disease
　　Chronic lung disease
　　Haemoglobin variant with increased oxygen affinity
　Erythropoietin inappropriately increased
　　Renal disease: hypernephroma, renal cyst, hydronephrosis
　　Uterine myoma
　Other tumours, e.g. hepatocellular carcinoma, bronchial carcinoma

Relative (spurious) polycythaemia
　Plasma volume depletion
　Stress ('pseudo-polycythaemia')
　Dehydration
　Diuretic therapy

PRV, polycythaemia rubra vera

Table 26.3 Causes of marrow fibrosis

Primary

Secondary
　Metastatic cancer
　Acute leukaemia, especially megakaryocytic
　Myelodysplasia
　Hairy cell leukaemia
　Connective tissue disease, e.g. systemic lupus erythematosus
　Other, e.g. tuberculosis

27 Myeloproliferative disorders II: polycythaemia rubra vera

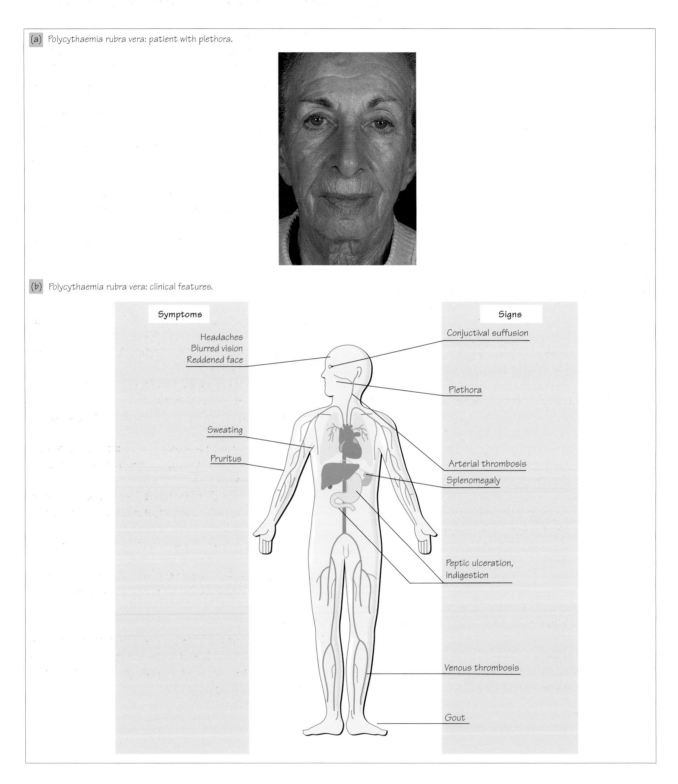

(a) Polycythaemia rubra vera: patient with plethora.

(b) Polycythaemia rubra vera: clinical features.

Symptoms	Signs
Headaches	Conjuctival suffusion
Blurred vision	Plethora
Reddened face	Arterial thrombosis
Sweating	Splenomegaly
Pruritus	Peptic ulceration, indigestion
	Venous thrombosis
	Gout

Polycythaemia rubra vera

Aetiology and pathophysiology

Polycythaemia rubra vera (PRV) is a primary neoplastic disorder in which bone marrow erythropoiesis is increased, usually accompanied by increased thrombopoiesis and granulopoiesis. Serum erythropoietin (EPO) levels are normal or low. The JAK 2 gene product is a tyrosine kinase which has a key role in signal transduction (see Chapter 1). A mutation is present in >95% of cases of PRV (and also in about 50% of cases with essential thrombocythaemia and myelofibrosis) which has the effect of amplifying the growth-promoting action of EPO. The mutation is usually heterozygous, but in a minority it is homozygous and has a more profound effect.

Clinical features
- PRV occurs equally in males and females, typically over 55 years of age.
- Raised red cell mass causes a ruddy complexion (Fig. 27a) and conjunctival suffusion; hyperviscosity may lead to headaches and visual disturbance.
- Thrombosis (e.g. deep vein thrombosis (DVT), Budd–Chiari syndrome, stroke) is also caused by hyperviscosity and increased platelets.
- Haemorrhage, especially gastrointestinal, may occur.
- Excess histamine secretion from basophils leads to increased gastric acid and peptic ulcer is frequent.
- Pruritus, typically after a hot bath, and gout, caused by increased uric acid production, also occur frequently.
- Enlarged spleen is found in 75% of patients and distinguishes PRV from other causes of polycythaemia (Fig. 27b).
- Gout may occur due to increased cell turnover.

Laboratory features
- Raised haematocrit, haemoglobin concentration, red cell count and RCM.
- Seventy five per cent of patients have raised white cells (neutrophil leucocytosis) and/or platelets.
- JAK 2 mutation Val617Phe in >95% of patients; rare cases show other mutations in JAK 2.
- Serum uric acid is usually raised.
- Serum LD normal or slightly raised
- EPO usually low
- Bone marrow is hypercellular with prominent megakaryocytes, iron stores are depleted because of excessive iron utilization, and the trephine biopsy may show mildly increased reticulin.
- Abdominal ultrasound excludes renal disease and assesses spleen size.
- Culture of peripheral blood cells shows spontaneous formation of erythroid colonies in the absence of exogenous EPO.

Differential diagnosis
The JAK 2 mutation is absent in all other forms of polycythaemia. Secondary or reactive polycythaemia may occur in conditions where arterial oxygen saturation is reduced, leading to a physiological rise in serum EPO, or when EPO levels are inappropriately raised (e.g. caused by secretion of EPO by a renal neoplasm).

Spurious (pseudo) polycythaemia arises when plasma volume is reduced by dehydration, vomiting or diuretic therapy. A common form occurs particularly in some young male adults, especially smokers, and particularly is associated with stress, increased vasomotor tone and hypertension (Gaisböck's syndrome). The white cell and platelet counts are normal, as is the bone marrow and RCM. If the packed cell volume (PCV) is over 0.50, it is treated by venesections; patients should reduce weight, stop smoking, moderate alcohol intake and avoid diuretics.

The following additional tests are occasionally required.
- Chest X-ray; arterial blood gas analysis to exclude lung disease.
- Haemoglobin oxygen dissociation curve to identify a variant haemoglobin with increased oxygen affinity.
- Serum EPO assay.

Treatment
- Thrombosis is the main cause of morbidity and mortality and its incidence can be reduced by maintaining the PCV below 0.45 and platelets below 600×10^9/L. Aspirin (75 mg daily) is used to inhibit platelet function.
- Multiple venesections are used initially to lower the PCV and in some cases for long-term treatment.
- Chemotherapy (e.g. oral hydroxycarbamide) is also usually required.
- ^{32}P is a β-emitter which is taken up and concentrated by bone and may be used to give prolonged myelosuppression (about 2 yr) in older patients.
- Busulphan may be given orally. It has a more prolonged action than hydroxycarbamide and more side effects and is now rarely used.
- A proton pump inhibitor is used for patients with indigestion.
- Allopurinol is used to prevent hyperuricaemia.
- Specific JAK 2 inhibiting drugs are in clinical trial.

Prognosis
Median survival is about 16 years. Up to 30% of patients develop myelofibrosis (see below). Acute myeloid leukaemia occurs in up to 5% of patients, probably increased in patients treated with a ^{32}P but not by hydroxycarbamide.

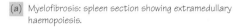
(a) Myelofibrosis: spleen section showing extramedullary haemopoiesis.

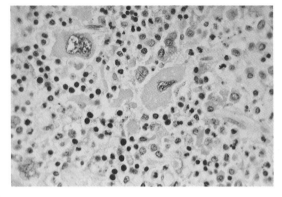

(b) Myelofibrosis: peripheral blood film showing aniso/poikilocytosis, teardrop forms and giant platelets.

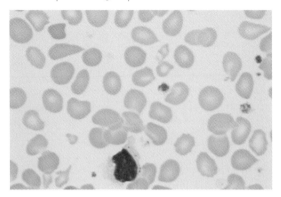

(c) Myelofibrosis: bone marrow biopsy showing increased cellularity and large numbers of megakaryocytes.

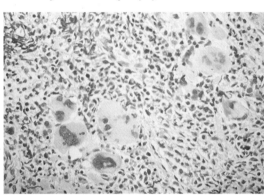

(d) Myelofibrosis: bone marrow biopsy (reticulin stain) showing increased reticulin.

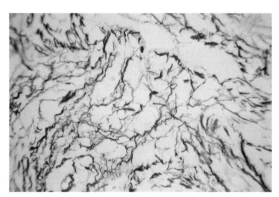

Essential thrombocythaemia

Essential thrombocythaemia (ET) is defined as persistent elevation of the peripheral blood platelet count as a result of increased marrow production in the absence of a systemic cause for thrombocytosis (Table 26.2).

Aetiology and pathophysiology

Similar to polycythaemia rubra vera (PRV), distinction between the two conditions is not exact. ET occurs more frequently in younger adults than PRV.

Clinical features

• Thrombosis, both arterial (peripheral vessels with gangrene of toes, cerebral, coronary and mesenteric arteries) and ve-nous (e.g. Budd–Chiari syndrome, deep vein thrombosis). Headaches, visual disturbance and peripheral vascular disease occur.

• At least 20% of patients are asymptomatic and detected as an incidental finding.

• Excessive haemorrhage may occur spontaneously or after trauma or surgery.

• Pruritus and sweating are uncommon.

• Splenomegaly in about 30% of patients; in others, the spleen is atrophied because of infarction.

Laboratory features

• Platelet count is persistently raised and often >1000 × 10⁹/L, raised red cell and/or white cell count is present in about 30%.

- Blood film shows platelet anisocytosis with circulating megakaryocyte fragments. Autoinfarction of the spleen causes changes in red cells (target cells, Howell–Jolly bodies).
- The JAK 2 mutation is present in about 50% of cases. In a few, this is homozygous and these tend to be more severe.
- Serum uric acid is often raised, serum LD may be raised.
- Bone marrow is hypercellular with increased numbers of megakaryocytes, often in aggregates.
- Defective platelet function, especially defective aggregation in response to adenosine diphosphate (ADP) and adrenaline, may help to distinguish primary from reactive thrombocythaemia.

Treatment
- Chemotherapy: hydroxycarbamide is used to maintain the platelet count below 400×10^9/L.
- α-Interferon may be used in younger subjects but needs injections and has side effects (flu like).
- Anagrelide is also effective but may cause cardiovascular or gastrointestinal side effects.
- Aspirin (75 mg daily), except in those with haemorrhage.
- JAK 2 inhibitors are in clinical trial.

Prognosis
Median survival is more than 20 years; thrombosis and haemorrhage are the main causes of morbidity and mortality. Transformation to acute myeloid leukaemia may occur.

Myelofibrosis
Myelofibrosis (myelosclerosis, agnogenic myeloid metaplasia) is characterized by splenomegaly, extramedullary haemopoiesis, a leucoerythroblastic blood picture and replacement of bone marrow by collagen fibrosis. It must be distinguished from secondary causes of marrow fibrosis (Table 26.3).

Aetiology and pathophysiology
Primary defect is within the haemopoietic stem cell; fibrosis results from a reactive non-neoplastic proliferation of marrow stromal cells. One-third patients have a preceding history of PRV or ET.

Clinical features
- Sexes affected equally; age of onset rarely below 50 years.
- Massive splenomegaly may lead to left hypochondrial pain (Fig. 28a).
- Fever, weight loss, pruritus, hepatomegaly and night sweats are frequent; gout, bone and joint pain are less common.
- Abdominal swelling, ascites and bleeding from oesophageal varices occur, caused by portal hypertension, in late stages.

Laboratory features
- Normochromic normocytic anaemia.
- Leucocytosis and thrombocytosis with circulating megakaryocyte fragments occur early, and later the leucopenia and thrombocytopenia.
- Blood film: red cell poikilocytosis with teardrop forms (Fig. 28b) and circulating red cell and white cell precursors (leucoerythroblastic picture).
- The JAK 2 mutation is present in about 50% of cases.
- Serum LDH is raised more than in PRV or ET.
- Liver function tests are often abnormal because of extramedullary haemopoiesis.
- Bone marrow aspiration is usually unsuccessful ('dry tap'); the trephine biopsy shows increased cellularity, increased megakaryocytes and fibrosis (Figs. 28c–d).

Treatment
- Chemotherapy (e.g. hydroxycarbamide) for patients with hypermetabolism and myeloproliferation.
- Thalidomide improves marrow function and reduces spleen size in about a third of cases; trials are in progress with the thalidomide derivative, lenalidomide.
- Supportive therapy with red cell transfusions, folic acid and occasionally platelet transfusions. Iron chelation may be needed.
- Allopurinol to prevent hyperuricaemia and gout.
- Splenectomy or splenic irradiation to reduce symptoms from splenomegaly, anaemia or thrombocytopenia (selected patients).
- Allogeneic stem cell transplantation has cured some younger patients (<60 yr).
- JAK 2 inhibitors are in clinical trial.

Prognosis
Median survival is about 5 years; acute leukaemia occurs in about 20%.

29 Chronic lymphocytic leukaemia

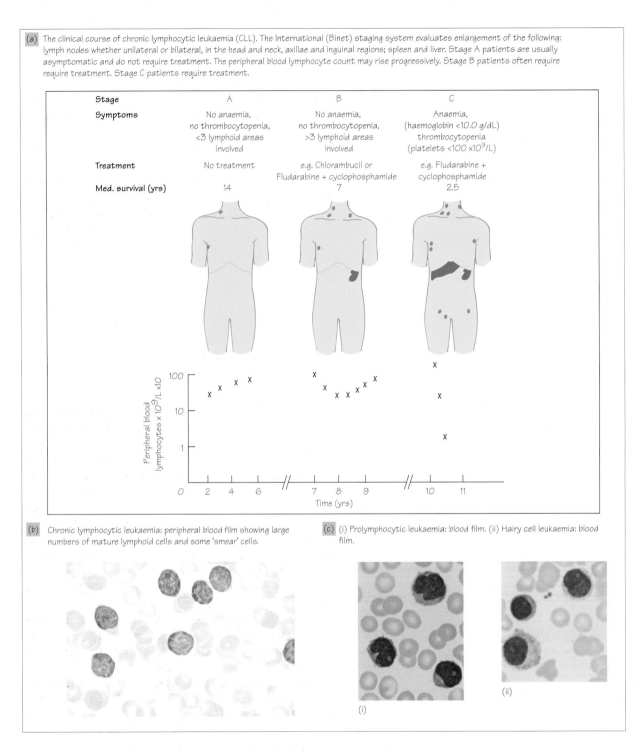

(a) The clinical course of chronic lymphocytic leukaemia (CLL). The International (Binet) staging system evaluates enlargement of the following: lymph nodes whether unilateral or bilateral, in the head and neck, axillae and inguinal regions; spleen and liver. Stage A patients are usually asymptomatic and do not require treatment. The peripheral blood lymphocyte count may rise progressively. Stage B patients often require require treatment. Stage C patients require treatment.

Stage	A	B	C
Symptoms	No anaemia, no thrombocytopenia, <3 lymphoid areas involved	No anaemia, no thrombocytopenia, >3 lymphoid areas involved	Anaemia, (haemoglobin <10.0 g/dL) thrombocytopenia (platelets <100 ×10⁹/L)
Treatment	No treatment	e.g. Chlorambucil or Fludarabine + cyclophosphamide	e.g. Fludarabine + cyclophosphamide
Med. survival (yrs)	14	7	2.5

(b) Chronic lymphocytic leukaemia: peripheral blood film showing large numbers of mature lymphoid cells and some 'smear' cells.

(c) (i) Prolymphocytic leukaemia: blood film. (ii) Hairy cell leukaemia: blood film.

(i)

(ii)

Chronic lymphocytic leukaemia (CLL) is a B-cell clonal lymphoproliferative disease in which lymphocytes accumulate in the blood, bone marrow and often in the lymph nodes and spleen (absolute lymphocyte count >5.0 × 10⁹/L). A disease of older patients (peak age 72), it is the commonest leukaemia in Western countries (over 70 new cases per million population per year in the UK, male/female ratio 2:1) but is rare in Asia.

Aetiology and pathophysiology

The cause is unknown. Commonest chromosome changes are trisomy 12, a 13q deletion and deletions of 11q including the ataxia telangiectasia gene. Oncogene mutations or deletions occur, which may prevent cells from undergoing apoptosis. The 13q deletion is thought to eliminate expression of several micro-RNAs (see p. 49). Mutations or deletions of the P53 gene

Haematology at a Glance, 3e. By A. Mehta and V. Hoffbrand. Published 2009 by Blackwell Publishing. ISBN 978-1-4051-7970-6.

Table 29.1 Prognostic features of CLL

	Favourable	Unfavourable
Sex	Female	Male
Stage	A	B, C
Lymphocyte doubling time	>1 yr	<6 mo
Auto immune Haemolytic anaemia	absent	present
ZAP-70	Negative	Positive
CD 38	Negative	Positive
Somatic mutation at IgH locus	Mutated	Germline
Cytogenetics	13q deletion	Trisomy 12 P53 deletions

(chromosome 17) may be present initially or develop during the cause of the disease. They have adverse prognostic significance.

Clinical features

Stage depends on clinical and laboratory findings (Fig. 29a).
- Most cases (Stage A) are symptomless and diagnosed on routine blood test.
- Presenting features include lymphadenopathy (typically symmetrical, painless and discrete), night sweats, loss of weight, symptoms of bone marrow failure.
- Spleen is often moderately enlarged.
- Hypogammaglobulinaemia and reduced cell-mediated immunity predispose to bacterial and viral infection.
- Autoimmune haemolytic anaemia in 15–25% of cases.

Laboratory findings

- Increased peripheral blood lymphocytes (Fig. 29b usually 5–30×10^9/L at presentation) which are B cells (CD19, CD22 but also CD5 positive).
- They have weak expression of surface IgM which is monoclonal (expressing only κ or only λ light chains).
- Serum immunoglobulins are depressed.
- Anaemia and thrombocytopenia may occur due to marrow infiltration or as a result of autoantibodies.
- Expression of a protein kinase ZAP-70 and CD38 are increased in some (poorer prognostic) cases.
- Degree of somatic mutation in IgH immunoglobulin gene relates to prognosis (Table 29.1). Germline (unmutated) cases are derived from pre-germinal centre B cells and have a worse prognosis.
- Cytogenetic changes – these have been described above

Course and prognosis

Many patients present at an early stage and subsequently remain stationary or progress very slowly. Others present with late-stage disease. Some patients never need treatment, whilst in others the disease follows an aggressive course. Local lymphoblastic transformation (Richter's syndrome) may be a terminal event. The natural history correlates with the maturity of the cell of origin, post-germinal centre (good) or pre-germinal centre (bad).

Treatment

- Observation only for asymptomatic Stage A patients.
- The purine analogue fludarabine is valuable in combination with cyclophosphamide (FC) as initial or subsequent therapy. Trials of FC with rituximab are in progress.
- Oral chlorambucil gives fewer complete responses than FC, but overall survival may be similar.
- Corticosteroids for bone marrow failure due to infiltration and for autoimmune haemolytic anaemia or thrombocytopenia.
- Combination chemotherapy e.g. CHOP (see Chapter 34).
- Monoclonal antibodies, rituximab (anti-CD20) or Alemtuzumab (anti-CD52) may be used in late-stage disease. Rituximab may be valuable if used earlier and can also be used to treat autoimmune cytopenias.
- Support care (Chapter 49).
- Splenectomy or splenic irradiation is useful if the spleen is large and causes local symptoms or hypersplenism.
- Allogeneic stem cell transplantation may cure some younger patients but has a high mortality.

Variants of CLL

Prolymphocytic leukaemia (PLL) (Fig. 29c(i)) resembles CLL but usually occurs in older (>70 yr) patients, the white cell count is high and responds poorly to treatment.

Hairy cell leukaemia (HCL) (Fig. 29c(ii)) is rare (male/female ratio of 4:1, peak age of 55 yr), presents with splenomegaly and pancytopenia. 'Hairy cells' are present in bone marrow and blood. Infections are frequent. They are B cells expressing CD19 and CD20 but also CD11c and CD103, which stain for tartrate-resistant acid phosphatase. Effective treatments include 2-chlorodeoxyadenosine deoxycoformycin, rituximab, interferon-α and splenectomy.

T-cell variant of PLL is much rarer than B-cell type and more aggressive.

Adult T-cell leukaemia/lymphoma is a disease caused by HTLV-1 infection mainly in the Caribbean and Japan. Hypercalcaemia, skin involvement and widespread lymphadenopathy are typical. The prognosis is poor.

Large granular lymphocyte leukaemia is a rare, chronic clonal disease characterized by a T-cell lymphocytosis, often with anaemia or neutropenia.

Leukaemia/lymphoma syndromes: Circulating lymphoma cells may occur in different non-Hodgkin lymphomas, e.g. follicular lymphoma, mantle cell lymphoma, lymphoplasmacytic lymphoma and adult T-cell leukaemia/lymphoma.

30 Multiple myeloma

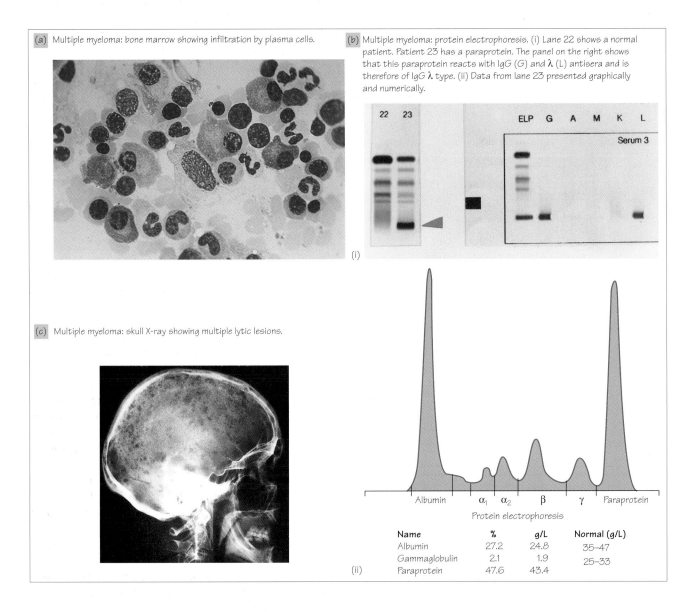

(a) Multiple myeloma: bone marrow showing infiltration by plasma cells.

(b) Multiple myeloma: protein electrophoresis. (i) Lane 22 shows a normal patient. Patient 23 has a paraprotein. The panel on the right shows that this paraprotein reacts with IgG (G) and λ (L) antisera and is therefore of IgG λ type. (ii) Data from lane 23 presented graphically and numerically.

(c) Multiple myeloma: skull X-ray showing multiple lytic lesions.

Name	%	g/L	Normal (g/L)
Albumin	27.2	24.8	35–47
Gammaglobulin	2.1	1.9	25–33
Paraprotein	47.6	43.4	

Multiple myeloma is a malignant disorder of plasma cells characterized by

1 a monoclonal paraprotein in serum and/or urine;
2 bone changes leading to pain and pathological features and
3 excess plasma cells in the bone marrow.

Incidence

Approximately 50 cases per million population; 15% of lymphoid malignancies; 2% of all malignancies; twice as common in black than white people; slightly more common in males than in females; median age at diagnosis 71 years.

Aetiology and pathogenesis

The aetiology is unknown. The cell of origin is probably a post-germinal centre B-lymphoid cell. The cells all secrete the same immunoglobulin (Ig) or Ig component, e.g. part of a heavy chain attached to a light chain or light chain (κ or λ). Rarely (<1%), the cells are non-secretory. Interleukin-6 (IL-6) from myeloma cells themselves or accessory cells promotes plasma cell growth. Tumour necrosis factor and IL-1 mediate bone resorption. Oncogene mutations (e.g. *ras*, p53, *myc*) and translocations to 14q occur. Cyclin D1 is often overexpressed. Chromosome 11 and 13q deletions generally imply a poor prognosis.

Clinical features

• Bone pain, especially lower backache, or pathological fracture due to skeletal involvement.
• Bone marrow failure due to marrow infiltration.
• Infection – lack of normal immunoglobulins (immune paresis) and neutropenia.

- Renal failure occurs in up to one-third patients and is caused by hypercalcaemia, infection, deposition of paraprotein or light chains, uric acid or amyloid.
- Amyloidosis may cause macroglossia, hepatosplenomegaly, cardiac or renal failure, carpal tunnel syndrome and autonomic neuropathy.

Laboratory features

- Anaemia is frequent, often with neutropenia and thrombocytopenia. Erythrocyte sedimentation rate often >100 mm/h.
- Blood film shows rouleaux with a bluish background staining, caused by the protein increase. Leucoerythroblastic picture may be present.
- Bone marrow shows >15% plasma cells, often with multinucleate and other abnormal forms (Fig. 30a) These cells are CD 138 positive.
- A paraprotein in serum and/or Bence Jones protein (light chains) in urine with suppression of normal serum immunoglobulins is usual (Fig. 30b).
- The paraprotein is IgG in 70%; IgA in 20%; IgM is uncommon; IgD and IgE are rare.
- Serum light chain (either κ or λ) increased.
- Serum β_2 microglobulin (β_2M) often raised and higher levels correlate with worse prognosis.
- X-rays, CT scan or MRI show lytic lesions typically in skull and axial skeleton and/or osteoporosis, often with pathological fractures (Fig. 30c). Occasional patients show localized plasma cell deposits, typically in the axial skeleton (multiple or solitary plasmacytoma).
- Prognostic data include haemoglobin level, serum levels of β_2M, serum creatinine, serum albumin and extent of skeletal disease.

Treatment

- Symptomless patients who are stable with normal blood counts and renal function, no skeletal disease and low levels of paraprotein warrant observation rather than therapy.
- Chemotherapy: initial treatment depends on age. In patients >65 years, induction is usually with melphalan, prednisolone and thalidomide.
- Most patients will reach a stable (plateau) phase (clinically well with near normal blood count, <5% plasma cells in bone marrow, stable paraprotein level) after – four to six cycles of treatment. This lasts 1–3 years.
- Younger patients (<65 yr) benefit from intensive induction with courses of e.g. cyclophosphamide, dexamethasone and thalidomide followed by high-dose chemotherapy, e.g. with high-dose melphalan and autologous peripheral blood stem cell transplant.

- Most patients relapse and median survival is 4–6 years from diagnosis. Relapsed cases may be retreated with newer drugs, other combinations, e.g. idarubicin and dexamethasone, may even respond to initial therapy.
- New drug therapies include thalidomide derivatives, e.g. lenalidomide and the proteosome inhibitor bortezomib (Velcade).
- Radiotherapy is helpful in relieving pain from localized skeletal disease; hemi-body radiotherapy may help to control systemic disease.
- Allogeneic stem cell transplant may be curative if applied to selected younger (<50 yr) patients early in the course of the disease but procedure-related mortality rate is high.
- Supportive care includes hydration to prevent/treat renal failure, allopurinol to prevent hyperuricaemia, hydration, steroids and bisphosphonates for hypercalcaemia, antibiotics and blood components. Bisphosphonates (e.g. oral sodium clodronate, or intravenous pamidronate or zoledronate) are useful in reducing skeletal complications and may improve survival. Surgery may be required for complications (e.g. pathological fracture, spinal cord compression). Plasma exchange is helpful in reducing the paraprotein level quickly.

Related disorders

Benign monoclonal gammopathy (also termed monoclonal gammopathy of undetermined significance, MGUS) is an indolent disorder, more common than myeloma and characterized by a low (<25 g/L) and stationary serum level of paraprotein, no reduction in normal immunoglobulins, no or mild increase in one or other light chain, absence of skeletal abnormalities and of Bence Jones protein and less than 10% plasma cells in the marrow. It may progress slowly to myeloma or lymphoma in approximately 1% of patients per year of follow-up.

Primary amyloidosis also shows less than 10% marrow plasma cells and no skeletal lesions, but Bence Jones protein and low-level serum paraprotein with an increase in serum κ or λ light chain may occur (see p. 66). Treatment as for myeloma may be beneficial.

Solitary plasmacytoma may occur in bone or in soft tissues, a low level of serum paraprotein may occur and some cases later develop myeloma.

Lymphoplasmacytic lymphoma (Waldenström's macroglobulinaemia) (see Chapter 33) is a chronic lymphoproliferative disorder (median age >70 yr) associated with an IgM paraprotein. Hyperviscosity is common and may cause visual disturbance, central nervous system changes (confusion, impaired conscious level) and headache. Cells resembling plasma cells and lymphocytes are present in the marrow and often in the spleen and lymph nodes.

Plasma cell leukaemia is an aggressive disorder in which large numbers of plasma cells circulate. The prognosis is poor.

(a) Hodgkin lymphoma: lymph node biopsy showing a Reed–Sternberg cell (multinucleate cell) (arrows).

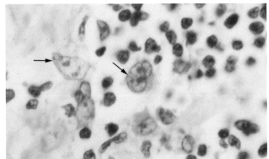

(b) Hodgkin lymphoma: varicella zoster infection.

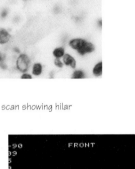

(c) Hodgkin lymphoma: (i) chest X-ray and (ii) CT scan showing hilar lymphadenopathy.

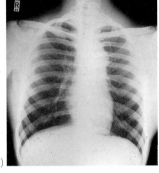

(i)   (ii)

(d) Hodgkin lymphoma: clinical features and staging. Stage I: involvement of a single lymph node region or structure; stage II: involvement of two or more lymph node regions on the same side of the diaphragm; stage III: involvement of lymph node regions or structures on both sides of the diaphragm; stage IV: involvement of other organs, e.g. liver, bone marrow, CNS. A: no symptoms; B: fever, night sweats, weight loss >10% in preceding 6 months; X: bulky disease; >1/3 widening of mediastinum; 10-cm max dimension of nodal mass; E: extralymphoid disease (e.g. in lung, skin).

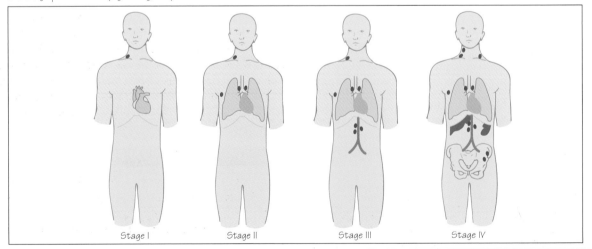

Stage I   Stage II   Stage III   Stage IV

Lymphoma is a clonal neoplastic proliferation of lymphoid cells originating in lymph nodes or other lymphoid tissue. It is a heterogeneous group of disorders, divided into Hodgkin lymphoma (HL) and non-Hodgkin lymphoma (NHL). Approximately 200 new cases per million population are diagnosed each year, with a ratio of NHL/HL of approximately 6:1; the incidence is rising. This chapter deals with HL. NHL is discussed in Chapters 32–34.

Aetiology and epidemiology

HL is more prevalent in males than in females (M/F ratio is 1.5–2.0:1) and has a peak incidence in age range of 15–40 years. The cause is not known, but Epstein–Barr virus (EBV) infection may be a cofactor.

Histological classification (Table 31.1)

This is well defined and of prognostic significance (see Table 31.1). Reed–Sternberg (RS) cells are characteristic of HL (Fig. 31a) but are usually outnumbered by a nonmalignant reactive infiltrate of eosinophils, plasma cells, lymphocytes and histiocytes. HL is of B-cell origin. Prognosis for lymphocyte-rich HL is favourable, whereas lymphocyte-depleted HL is less favourable.

Clinical features

- Lymphadenopathy (typically cervical and painless) is the characteristic presentation. The nodes often fluctuate in size, and alcohol ingestion may precipitate pain.
- Hepatic and splenic enlargement may occur.
- Systemic symptoms (fever, weight loss, pruritus and drenching night sweats) occur in 25%.
- Extranodal disease is uncommon but lung, central nervous system, skin and bone involvement may occur.
- Infection caused by defective cell-mediated/humoral immunity (Fig. 31b).

Laboratory features

- Anaemia (normochromic, normocytic).
- Leucocytosis (occasionally eosinophilia).
- Leucoerythroblastic blood film.
- Raised erythrocyte sedimentation rate
- Raised lactate dehydrogenase – useful as prognostic marker and for monitoring response,
- Abnormal liver function tests.

Staging

Staging influences both treatment and prognosis. Clinical staging with careful physical examination is followed by cervical, thoracic, abdominal and pelvic CT, PET/CT or MRI scanning (Fig. 31c). PET/CT is indicated to exclude distant disease in

Table 31.1 Histological classification of Hodgkin lymphoma

Hodgkin lymphoma
Nodular lymphocyte predominant Hodgkin lymphoma
Classical Hodgkin lymphoma
    Nodular sclerosis classical Hodgkin lymphoma
    Lymphocyte-rich classical Hodgkin lymphoma
    Mixed cellularity classical Hodgkin lymphoma
    Lymphocyte-depleted classical Hodgkin lymphoma

patients otherwise classified as stage IA or IIA and to receive radiotherapy. Bone marrow aspirate and trephine are performed to detect marrow involvement. The most commonly used staging system is the Cotswold classification (Fig. 31d).

Treatment

This depends principally on stage.
- Radiotherapy alone may be used for patients with clinical or pathological stage IA or IIA disease with favourable histology.
- Advanced (stages IB, IIB, III and IV) Hodgkin disease should be treated with combination chemotherapy (CCT) using one of the standard regimes (e.g. six cycles of adriamycin, bleomycin, vinblastine and dacarbazine, ABVD). PET/CT scan after two courses can be used to determine whether or not to intensify therapy.
- For bulky mediastinal disease, especially common in young females with nodular sclerosing HL, chemotherapy followed by deep X-ray therapy (DXT) (combined modality therapy) may be given and local DXT may be needed for other sites of bulky or resistant disease.

For complications of treatment, see Chapter 49.

Relapsed disease

Patients who relapse following DXT alone generally have a very good response to CCT (>80% complete remission (CR) rate). Patients initially treated with chemotherapy who relapse after a remission lasting more than 1 year are likely to achieve CR again, and up to 50% may be cured with CCT. However, patients relapsing within 1 year of initial therapy, or failing to achieve complete remission, have a poorer prognosis and should be considered for high-dose therapy with stem cell rescue (see Chapter 48).

Prognosis

Stage is of paramount importance for HL. While >90% of stage I and II may be cured, the rate falls progressively to 50–70% of stage IV patients. Older patients generally do less well, as do those with lymphocyte-depleted histology or leucocytosis to $>15.0 \times 10^9$/L.

Lymphoma II: Non-Hodgkin lymphoma – aetiology and classification

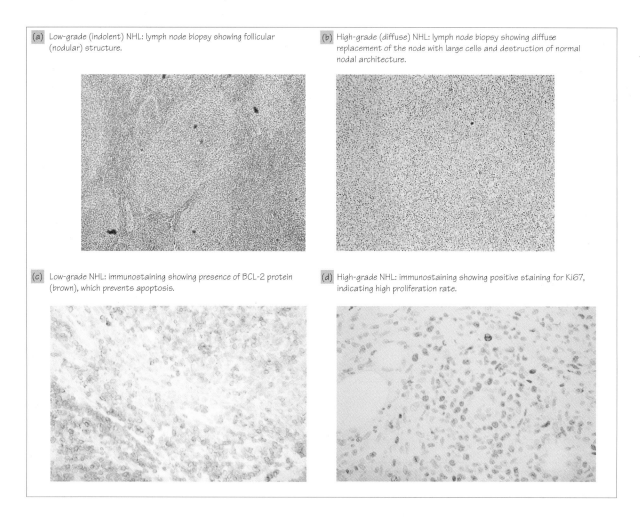

(a) Low-grade (indolent) NHL: lymph node biopsy showing follicular (nodular) structure.

(b) High-grade (diffuse) NHL: lymph node biopsy showing diffuse replacement of the node with large cells and destruction of normal nodal architecture.

(c) Low-grade NHL: immunostaining showing presence of BCL-2 protein (brown), which prevents apoptosis.

(d) High-grade NHL: immunostaining showing positive staining for Ki67, indicating high proliferation rate.

These diseases are divided into the more frequent B-cell types (85%) and the less common T-cell types (Table 32.1). The individual subtypes are characterized by their clinical and histological features, immunostaining and chromosome changes. The features of some of the more common types are briefly described in Chapter 33. Some of the general features are reviewed here.

Aetiology and epidemiology

Non-Hodgkin lymphoma (NHL) occurs at all ages, with indolent tumours being most common in the elderly. There is clonal expansion from a normal cell which is 'frozen' at a particular level of differentiation. Most NHLs are B-cell disorders. Environmental factors include abnormal response to viral infection, e.g. Epstein–Barr virus (EBV) in Burkitt's lymphoma (BL) and human T-cell leukaemia virus (HTLV-1) in adult T-cell leukaemia lymphoma (ATLL), or bacterial infection (e.g. chronic *Helicobactor pylori* infection in gastric lymphoma), or radiation or certain drugs (e.g. phenytoin). Autoimmune disease (e.g. Sjögren's syndrome, rheumatoid arthritis) and immune suppression (e.g. AIDS, post-transplant) also predispose to NHL. Chromosome translocations in NHL involving oncogenes and immunoglobulin genes include t(14;18) (follicular lymphoma (FL), BCL-2 oncogene) and t(8;14) (BL, MYC oncogene).

Clinical features

NHL is heterogeneous, but some common patterns occur.
• Lymphadenopathy is the most frequent clinical feature. It is often widely disseminated at presentation. The lymph nodes may be mainly superficial or deep and detected only by X-rays or scans.
• The spleen and less frequently the liver may be enlarged.
• Extranodal disease is more common than in Hodgkin lymphoma. Involvement of the gastrointestinal tract, central nervous system, skin (especially T-cell lymphomas), lung, thyroid and other organs occurs commonly in the various subtypes.
• Paraproteinaemia is usual in lymphoplasmacytic lymphoma.
• Particularly aggressive lymphomas include BL, some cases of diffuse large cell and anaplastic lymphoma, lymphomas associated with HIV infection and adult T-cell leukaemia/lymphoma (see Chapters 29 & 33).
FL and diffuse large B-cell lymphoma (DLBCL) are the two most common forms. Chronic lymphocytic leukaemia

Table 32.1 Non-Hodgkin lymphoma – WHO classification 2008 (simplified)

Mature B-cell neoplasms
CLL/SLL
B-cell PLL
Splenic marginal zone lymphoma
Hairy cell leukaemia
Lymphoplasmacytic lymphoma/Waldenstrom's
    macroglobulinaemia
Plasma cell myeloma
Extranodal marginal zone B-cell lymphoma of MALT lymphoma
Nodal marginal zone B-cell lymphoma
Follicular lymphoma
Mantle cell lymphoma
Diffuse large B-cell lymphoma
Burkitt's lymphoma/leukaemia
Post-transplant lymphoproliferative disorders. These are usually
    B-cell and may be polyclonal or clonal (lymphomas)

T-cell and NK-cell neoplasms
  Precursor T-cell neoplasms
    Precursor T-lymphoblastic lymphoma
    Blastic NK-cell lymphoma
  Mature T-cell and NK-cell neoplasms
    T-cell PLL
    T-cell large granular lymphocytic leukaemia
    Aggressive NK-cell leukaemia
    Adult T-cell leukaemia/lymphoma
    Extranodal NK/T-cell lymphoma, nasal type
    Enteropathy-type T-cell lymphoma
    Mycosis fungoides
    Sezary syndrome
    Primary cutaneous anaplastic large cell lymphoma
    Peripheral T-cell lymphoma, unspecified
    Angioimmunoblastic T-cell lymphoma
    Anaplastic large cell lymphoma

The World Health Organization (2008) classification (simplified) CLL, chronic lymphocytic leukaemia; HD, Hodgkin's disease; PLL, prolymphocytic leukaemia; SLL, small lymphocytic lymphoma; NK, natural killer; MALT, mucosa-associated lymphoid tissue

Table 32.2 Immunophenotype of mature B-cell neoplasms

	CD20/19a	CD10	CD5	Additional
CLL/small lympho-cytic lymphoma	+	−	+	
Hairy cell leukaemia	+	−	−	CD11c+ CD25c+ CD103+
Lymphoplasmacytic lymphoma	+	−	−	
Marginal zone lym-phoma of MALT	+	−	−	
Follicular lymphoma	+	+/−	−	Bcl-2+
Mantle cell lymphoma	+	−	+	CyctmD++
Diffuse large B-cell lymphoma	+	+/−	−	
Burkitt's lymphoma	+	+	−	

CLL, chronic lymphocytic leukaemia; MALT, mucosa-associated lymphoid tissue

- paraprotein and hypogammaglobulinaemia.
- Serum lactate dehydrogenase is raised in more aggressive forms.
- Raised β_2-microglobulin.
- Cytogenetics by conventional analysis or FISH may help to define.
- All patients will require histological diagnosis and immuno-histology is essential on node or bone marrow trephine biopsies to confirm the diagnosis of NHL and define the particular sub-type (Table 32.1).
- Gene array studies may be used to define prognostic groups within larger subtypes, e.g. diffuse large B cell, and FLs

Radiographic features

X-rays, CT scans, MRI and PET/CT scan are used for initial diagnosis, staging, for monitoring response to therapy (Fig. 34b) and for detecting low levels of disease when relapse is suspected.

Staging

The staging system is given in Fig. 31d. It is of less impor-tance than in HL, e.g. SLL or FL are often indolent and do not need treatment for many years despite presenting as stage IV, whereas aggressive lymphomas may proliferate rapidly locally and require urgent therapy.

Histological classification

NHL is classified as disease entities based on clinical, biologi-cal, cytogenetic and histological criteria. Membrane marker and molecular studies of NHL show most (>80%) to be derived from B cells (either follicle centre or from other zones in the lymph node), and the remainder are T cell or unclassified. Indolent NHL may evolve into aggressive disease (Figs 32a–d).

(CLL)-like indolent NHL (small lymphocytic lymphoma (SLL), FL), is more common in older patients (>60 yr) and is widely disseminated at presentation with superficial and deep lym-phadenopathy. It may only warrant observation, not treatment. Variants include some T-cell NHL (T-NHL) (e.g. mycosis fun-goides), which affect the skin, and splenic marginal zone lym-phoma predominantly causing splenomegaly.

Laboratory features

In addition to the changes seen in HL, NHL may cause:
- pancytopenia as a result of bone marrow involvement leading to bone marrow failure;
- peripheral blood lymphocytosis caused by the presence of lymphoma cells in the blood and

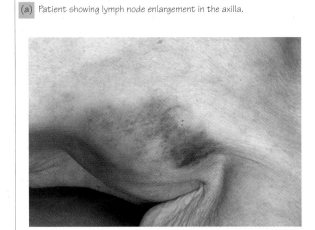

(a) Patient showing lymph node enlargement in the axilla.

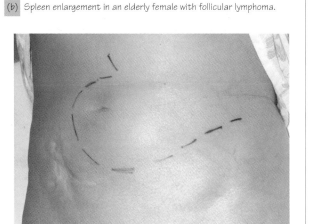

(b) Spleen enlargement in an elderly female with follicular lymphoma.

Low-grade B-cell lymphoma
Small lymphocytic lymphoma

This has similar clinical and laboratory features to chronic lymphocytic leukaemia but has no excess of circulating lymphocytes.

Lymphoplasmacytic lymphoma

This is a decrease in small lymphocytes, plasma cells and cells with lymphoplasmacytoid appearances. There is usually bone marrow, lymph node and spleen involvement and a paraprotein in serum which, in Waldenstrom's macroglobulinaemia, is IgM and likely to cause hyperviscosity.

Follicular lymphoma

This is the dominant form of low-grade lymphoma, mainly involving lymph nodes, usually widespread at diagnosis. The spleen and bone marrow are often involved and the disease may present as a primary skin tumour. The histology is characteristic of the nodes often being subdivided into three grades depending on the proportion of small and large cells in the neoplastic follicles. Over 80% of cells show the t(14;18) translocation with increased expression of Bcl-2, which inhibits cell apoptosis. The clinical course is often indolent for many years with therapy not being needed, but transformation to a more aggressive large cell lymphoma occurs in about one-third of cases when the prognosis is substantially reduced.

Marginal cell lymphoma

Splenic marginal cell lymphoma presents with an enlarged spleen often circulating monoclonal B lymphocytes (which may have villous appearance), autoimmune haemolysis and a paraprotein. Mucosa-associated lymphoid tissue (Malt) lymphomas occur particularly in the stomach associated with *Helicobacter*

pylori infection in early stages, and this may respond to antibiotic therapy. The disease may also involve the thyroid, lung or other soft tissues.

Mantle cell lymphoma

This usually presents as a low-grade lymphoma with a characteristic histological appearance, small cells with irregular, angular nuclei and a diagnostic cytogenetic change t(11;14), which leads to overexpression of cyclin D1. The prognosis is poor with a mean survival of only a few years.

High-grade lymphomas
Diffuse large cell lymphoma

This constitutes 30–40% of adult non-Hodgkin lymphoma in Western countries. The histological appearances vary but always include diffuse replacement of lymph node structure. Frequently presentation is extra nodal and central nervous system disease is frequent in HIV-infected patients. It may arise as a transformation of a small cell lymphoma. Despite its aggressive clinical course, it has a potential to be cured by courses of intensive chemotherapy. The disease may be divided into different prognostic groups by cytogenetic, immunohistological and gene array studies and by clinical parameters (Table 33.1).

Burkitt lymphoma

This is the most aggressive lymphoma which often presents at extranodal sites or as an acute leukaemia. It occurs in three clinical variants: *endemic BL* occurs in equational Africa and other tropical areas where malaria is frequent. It is common in children and presents with jaw or facial involvement in about 50% of patients with sites including soft tissue organs of the abdomen. *Sporadic BL* – this occurs throughout the world in both children and adults but accounts for only 1–2% of lymphomas. It typically presents with abdominal masses, rarely as

Table 33.1 International Prognostic Index (IPI)

	Adverse prognosis
Age	≥60 yr
Ann Arbor stage	III or IV
Serum LDH	Above normal
Number of extranodal sites	≥2
Performance status	ECOG2 or equivalent

acute leukaemia. *Immunodeficiency-associated BL* – this occurs mainly with HIV infection and may be a presenting feature. In all types, there is a high risk of central nervous system involvement and translocation of the oncogene C myc, usually due to the t(8;14) translocation. The individual cells are medium-sized basophilic cells with multiple cytoplasmic vacuoles. Histology gives a starry sky appearance due to pale staining macrophages which have ingested dying cells among the high-proliferating tumour cells.

Mature T-cell diseases

These account for only 10–15% of lymphomas. They are derived from post-thymic T cells and clinically vary widely from indolent to aggressive tumours with a poor prognosis. The WHO (2008) lists a large number of sub-varieties, the most frequent of which are listed in Table 32.1.

Peripheral T-cell lymphoma, unspecified, is the most common usually nodal, with skin and other extranodal sites frequently involved. Mycosis fungoides (MF) Sjögren's syndrome (SS) principally involve the skin; MF without blood involvement shows skin plaques or raised red patches and may become more aggressive with time. SS is more aggressive initially with tumour CD4$^+$ T cells in the blood and lymph node involvement.

Adult T-cell lymphoma/leukaemia occurs in the Caribbean, and other areas where the human T-cell lymphoproliferative virus (HTLV-1) is endemic. Typically, there is a skin rash, hypercalcaemia, a high white cell count due to leukaemic cells in the blood. Some cases present more as lymphomas with lymphadenopathy or with a chronic course. The neoplastic cells often slow polylobated nuclei (flower cells; see also Chapter 29).

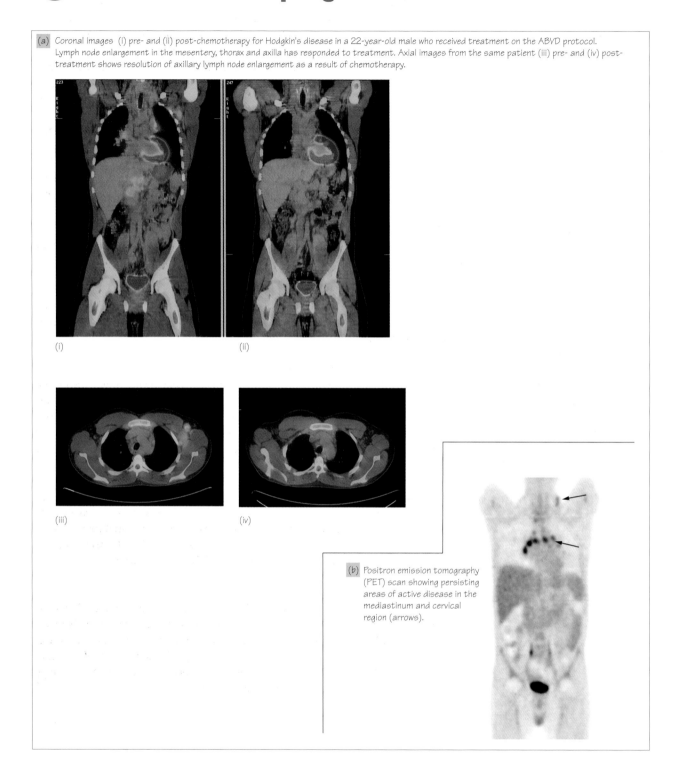

(a) Coronal images (i) pre- and (ii) post-chemotherapy for Hodgkin's disease in a 22-year-old male who received treatment on the ABVD protocol. Lymph node enlargement in the mesentery, thorax and axilla has responded to treatment. Axial images from the same patient (iii) pre- and (iv) post-treatment shows resolution of axillary lymph node enlargement as a result of chemotherapy.

(i)

(ii)

(iii)

(iv)

(b) Positron emission tomography (PET) scan showing persisting areas of active disease in the mediastinum and cervical region (arrows).

Treatment

This depends principally on clinical features, stage and accurate classification by histology including immunohistology and where appropriate cytogenetic or molecular studies. Paradoxically, aggressive tumours respond more dramatically to treatment and are more likely to be cured than indolent tumours. However, they are also rapidly progressive if untreated, frequently relapse and are associated with higher short- to medium-term mortality.

Aggressive

Localized (stage I or II) disease may be treated by deep X-ray therapy (DXT) with adjuvant combination chemotherapy (CCT) (e.g. three cycles of CHOP, a 21-day cycle of cyclophosphamide, hydroxydaunorubicin (Adriamycin), vincristine and prednisolone) with anti-CD20 monoclonal antibody (rituximab). Advanced stage aggressive non-Hodgkin lymphoma (NHL) is treated with CCT (usually CHOP–rituximab, up to complete remission plus at least two cycles); PET-CT scan is valuable to assess whether or not full remission has been achieved (Fig. 34). DXT to a single site of residual disease may be given. Diffuse large B-cell lymphoma (DLBCL) may be divided into better or worse prognosis based on immunohistology or gene arrays. More intensive therapy is considered for those with a worse prognosis.

Patients with B- or T-lymphoblastic lymphoma are best treated as for acute lymphoblastic leukaemia; such patients are candidates for allogeneic stem cell transplantation (see Chapter 48). Patients with Burkitt's lymphoma are treated as patients with mature B-cell acute lymphoblastic leukaemia with a different protocol using multiple drugs and incorporating high doses of drugs, e.g. methotrexate and cytosine arabinoside to penetrate the central nervous system (CNS). For HIV-positive patients, treatment of the viral infection with highly active antiretroviral therapy (HAART) is also given. Treatment of T-cell NHL to that for B-cell tumours is similar except that rituximab is not used. Tumour lysis syndrome protocols are needed with initial therapy for bulky DLBCL and Burkitt's lymphoma.

Patients with CNS disease are treated with protocols to include high-dose methotrexate and/or cytosine arabinoside aimed at penetrating the blood–brain barrier, with or without CNS radiotherapy. Intrathecal therapy is given for patients with all forms of aggressive lymphoma with a high risk of CNS disease.

Indolent

Asymptomatic patients, e.g. follicular lymphoma or small cell lymphocytic lymphoma, may be followed closely without therapy for months or even years. When treatment is required, options include single agent chemotherapy (e.g. oral chlorambucil) and CCT, e.g. cyclophosphamide, vincristine, prednisolone (CVP) with rituximab. Plasmapheresis may be needed to treat hyperviscosity in Waldenstrom's macroglobulinaemia. The relapse rate is high. Trials of aggressive chemotherapy followed by allogeneic stem cell transplantation are in progress for younger patients, particularly at first relapse. If an indolent tumour transforms to a high grade, intensive therapy with or without DXT is indicated, possibly with some form of stem cell transplantation.

Mantle cell lymphoma, despite its similarities to chronic lymphocytic leukaemia and small cell lymphocytic lymphoma, has a poor prognosis and aggressive therapy combined in younger patients with some form of SCT is being tried. *Malt lymphomas* (see p. 72) are treated as indolent diseases. Antibiotic therapy to eliminate *Heliobacter pylori* is given in early gastric disease. *Splenic marginal zone lymphoma* responds best to splenectomy.

Mycosis fungoides is treated with skin-targeted therapies, e.g. PUVA, topical steroids, nitrogen mustard or vitamin D. Sezary's syndrome is also treated systemically, e.g. CHOP or anti-CD 52 (alemtuzumab).

Relapsed disease

Over 50% of NHL patients will relapse after initial therapy. Indolent NHL will typically respond to further single agent therapy or to CCT or radiotherapy. Relapsed aggressive NHL carries a poor prognosis but may respond to second-line CCT regimes followed by autologous or allogeneic stem cell transplantation.

New therapies

Monoclonal antibodies, e.g. alemtuzumab, some bound to one or other radioactive toxins, e.g. Zevalin (see Chapter 49). New chemotherapy regimes have been introduced incorporating fludarabine, mitoxantrone, thalidomide derivatives, 2-chlorodeoxy-adenosine (2-CDA) and bortezomib.

Prognosis

Prognosis in NHL is largely dependent on histology. The presence of bulky disease, multiple sites of extranodal involvement, age, performance status and laboratory parameters, such as lactate dehydrogenase level and β_2-microglobulin level, all influence prognosis (Table 33.1). Long-term side effects of therapy are considered in Chapter 49.

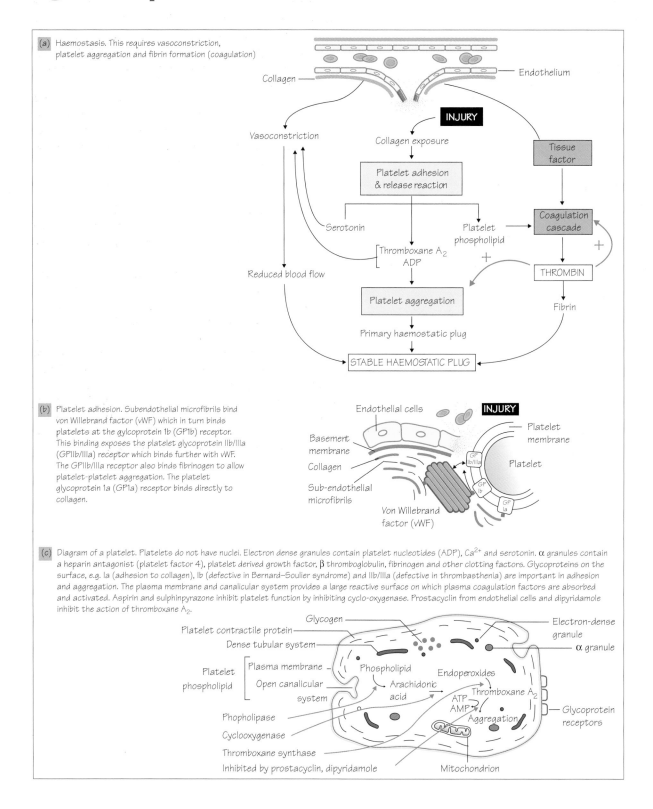

(a) Haemostasis. This requires vasoconstriction, platelet aggregation and fibrin formation (coagulation)

Collagen
Endothelium

INJURY

Vasoconstriction

Collagen exposure

Tissue factor

Platelet adhesion & release reaction

Serotonin

Platelet phospholipid

Coagulation cascade

Thromboxane A$_2$ ADP

Reduced blood flow

+

THROMBIN

+

Platelet aggregation

Fibrin

Primary haemostatic plug

STABLE HAEMOSTATIC PLUG

(b) Platelet adhesion. Subendothelial microfibrils bind von Willebrand factor (vWF) which in turn binds platelets at the gylcoprotein 1b (GP1b) receptor. This binding exposes the platelet glycoprotein IIb/IIIa (GPIIb/IIIa) receptor which binds further with vWF. The GPIIb/IIIa receptor also binds fibrinogen to allow platelet-platelet aggregation. The platelet glycoprotein 1a (GP1a) receptor binds directly to collagen.

Endothelial cells

INJURY

Basement membrane

Platelet membrane

Collagen

GP IIb/IIIa

Platelet

Sub-endothelial microfibrils

GP Ib

GP Ia

Von Willebrand factor (vWF)

(c) Diagram of a platelet. Platelets do not have nuclei. Electron dense granules contain platelet nucleotides (ADP), Ca^{2+} and serotonin. α granules contain a heparin antagonist (platelet factor 4), platelet derived growth factor, β thromboglobulin, fibrinogen and other clotting factors. Glycoproteins on the surface, e.g. Ia (adhesion to collagen), Ib (defective in Bernard–Soulier syndrome) and IIb/IIIa (defective in thrombasthenia) are important in adhesion and aggregation. The plasma membrane and canalicular system provides a large reactive surface on which plasma coagulation factors are absorbed and activated. Aspirin and sulphinpyrazone inhibit platelet function by inhibiting cyclo-oxygenase. Prostacyclin from endothelial cells and dipyridamole inhibit the action of thromboxane A$_2$.

Glycogen

Electron-dense granule

Platelet contractile protein

Dense tubular system

α granule

Plasma membrane

Phospholipid

Endoperoxides

Platelet phospholipid

Open canalicular system

Arachidonic acid

Thromboxane A$_2$

ATP
AMP

Glycoprotein receptors

Phopholipase

Aggregation

Cyclooxygenase

Thromboxane synthase

Inhibited by prostacyclin, dipyridamole

Mitochondrion

Haemostasis (Fig. 35a) is the process whereby haemorrhage following vascular injury is arrested. It depends on closely linked interaction between
- the vessel wall;
- platelets and
- coagulation factors.

The fibrinolytic system and inhibitors of coagulation ensure coagulation is limited to the site of injury.

Normal haemostasis is discussed in Chapters 35 and 36; disorders are considered in Chapters 37–39.

The vessel wall

The intact vessel wall has an important role in preventing haemostasis. Endothelial cells produce
- prostacyclin, which causes vasodilatation and inhibits platelet aggregation;
- protein C (PC) activator (thrombomodulin), which inhibits coagulation and
- tissue plasminogen activator (TPA), which activates fibrinolysis.

Injury to the vessel wall (a) activates membrane bound tissue factor, which initiates coagulation (Fig. 36a) and (b) exposes subendothelial connective tissue allowing binding of platelets to von Willebrand factor (vWF), a large, multimeric protein made by endothelial cells, which mediates platelet adhesion to endothelium and carries clotting factor VIII in plasma.

Platelets

Platelets have a large surface area onto which coagulation factors are adsorbed. Glycoproteins GPIb and IIb/IIIa allow attachment of platelets to vWF (Fig. 35b) and hence to endothelium. Collagen exposure and thrombin promote platelet aggregation and the platelet release reaction whereby platelets release their granule contents. Adenosine diphosphate (ADP) promotes platelet aggregation to form a primary haemostatic plug. Platelet prostaglandin synthesis is activated to form thromboxane A_2, which potentiates the platelet release reaction, promotes platelet aggregation and also has vasoconstrictor activity. Fibrin, produced by blood coagulation, binds to vWF and enmeshes the platelets to form a stable haemostatic plug. Activated platelets promote coagulation, as they have exposed phospholipid-binding sites which are involved in activation of factor X and prothrombin to thrombin in the coagulation cascade.

Thrombopoiesis

Megakaryocytes (see Fig. 1.1) are large multinucleated cells derived from haemopoietic stem cells. Platelets break off from the megakaryocyte cytoplasm and enter the peripheral blood. Thrombopoietin is produced mainly in the liver and stimulates megakaryocyte and platelet production by increasing differentiation of stem cells into megakaryocytes, increasing megakaryocyte numbers and increasing the number of divisions of megakaryocyte nuclei (ploidy). Platelets (Fig. 35c) are non-nucleated cells required for normal haemostasis. They circulate for 7–10 days. Their lifespan is reduced when there is increased platelet consumption (thrombosis, infection and splenic enlargement). Platelets appear in peripheral blood films as granular basophilic forms with a mean diameter of 1–2 μm. The normal concentration is 140–400×10^9/L; a lower number is found in neonates (100–300×10^9/L) and among certain racial populations, e.g. in Southern Europe or the Middle East.

Normal haemostasis II: coagulation factors and fibrinolysis

(a) The coagulation pathway. Injury initiates release of tissue factor (TF) which binds and activates factor VII. The TF VIIa complex activates factors X and IX; the activity of the TF VIIa complex is inhibited by TF pathway inhibitor (TFPI). The VIIIa–IXa complex amplifies Xa production from X. Thrombin is generated from prothrombin by the action of Xa–Va complex and this leads to fibrin formation. Thrombin also (i) activates FXI leading to increased FIXa production; (ii) cleaves FVIII from its carrier protein vWF activating FVIII; (iii) activates FV to FVa; and (iv) activates FXIII to XIIIa, which stabilizes the fibrin clot. Note that (i) TFPI inhibits TF/VIIa, Xa; (ii) Activated PC (APC) and PS inhibit Va, VIIIa; and (iii) antithrombin inhibits thrombin, Xa, IXa. Extrinsic pathway, Factor VII. Intrinsic pathway, Factors XI, IX, VIII. Common pathway, Factors X, V, II, fibrinogen.

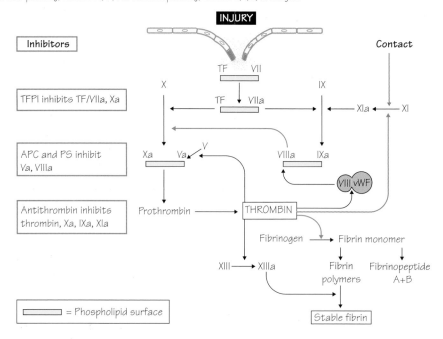

(b) Fibrinolysis. Injury causes release of TPA and UPA which, together with activated components from coagulation pathway and protein C, activate plasminogen to plasmin. Plasmin acts on insoluble fibrin to form a series of soluble products (fragments). Note that (i) plasminogen activator inhibitor inhibits activation of plasminogen; and (ii) α_2 antiplasmin and α_2 macroglobulin inhibit action of plasmin.

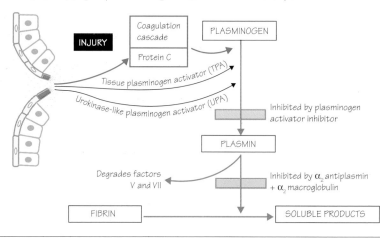

Coagulation factors

The proteins of the coagulation cascade are proenzymes (serine proteases) and procofactors, which are activated sequentially (Fig. 36a). The cascade has been divided on the basis of laboratory tests into intrinsic, extrinsic and common pathways. This division is useful in understanding results of in vitro coagulation tests. In vivo, however, these pathways are closely interlinked.

Coagulation begins when tissue factor is activated on the surface of injured cells and binds and activates factor VII; the complex activates factor X to Xa but also factor IX which, with cofactor VIII, substantially amplifies activation of factor X to Xa.

Platelets accelerate the coagulation process by providing membrane phospholipid. The complex of Xa and Va, activated from factor V by thrombin, acts on prothrombin (factor II) to

Table 36.1 Laboratory tests of coagulation

Screening test (normal range)	Abnormalities indicated (prolonged abnormal)	Most common cause of disorder
Prothrombin time (PT) (10–14 s)	Extrinsic and common coagulation pathways Deficiency/inhibition of factor VII, factors X, V, II and fibrinogen	Liver disease, warfarin therapy, DIC
Activated partial thromboplastin time (APTT or PTTK) (30–40 s)	Intrinsic and common coagulation pathways Deficiency/inhibition of one or more of factors XII, IX, VIII, X, V, II and fibrinogen	Liver disease, heparin therapy, haemophilia A and B, DIC
Thrombin time (14–16 s)	Deficiency or abnormality of fibrinogen; inhibition of thrombin by heparin or FDPs	DIC, heparin therapy, fibrinolytic
Fibrin degradation products (<10 mg/mL)	Accelerated destruction of fibrinogen	DIC
Platelet aggregation tests	Abnormal platelet function	Drugs (e.g. aspirin), uraemia, von Willebrand's disease.
Euglobulin clot lysis time	Fibrinolytic pathway defect	Smoking
Bleeding time (now largely replaced by PFA-100 test) (see text)	Platelet functional defect or thrombocytopenia	Drugs (aspirin), Von Willebrand's disease

DIC, disseminated intravascular coagulation; FDP, fibrin degradation product

generate thrombin. Thrombin then converts fibrinogen into fibrin monomers, with release of fibrinopeptides A and B. The monomers combine to form a fibrin polymer clot. Factor XIII cross-links the polymer to form a more stable clot.

Thrombin has a number of key roles in the coagulation process.

1 It converts plasma fibrinogen into fibrin.
2 It amplifies coagulation by (a) activating factor XI which increases IXa production, (b) cleaving factor VIII from its carrier molecule vWF to activate it and augment Xa production by the IXa–VIIIa complex and (c) activating factor V to factor Va.
3 It also activates factor XIII to factor XIIIa, which stabilizes the fibrin clot.
4 It potentiates platelet aggregation.
5 It binds to thrombomodulin on the endothelial cell surface to form a complex which activates protein C, which is involved in inhibiting coagulation.

Coagulation inhibitory factors

These inhibit the coagulation cascade and ensure the action of thrombin is limited to the site of injury.
• Antithrombin inactivates serine proteases, principally factor Xa and thrombin. Heparin activates antithrombin.
• Proteins C and S are vitamin K-dependent proteins made in the liver. Protein C is activated via a thrombin–thrombomodulin complex (Fig. 36b) and, like protein S, inhibits coagulation by inactivating factors Va and VIIIa; it also enhances fibrinolysis by inactivating the tissue plasmogen activator (TPA) inhibitor (see Fig. 36b).

• Tissue factor pathway inhibitor inhibits the main in vivo coagulation pathway by inhibiting factor VIIa and Xa.

The fibrinolytic pathway (Fig. 36b)

Fibrinolysis is the process whereby fibrin is degraded by plasmin. A circulating pro-enzyme, plasminogen, may be activated to plasmin:
• following injury, by TPA released from damaged or activated cells or
• by exogenous agents, e.g. streptokinase, or by therapeutic TPA or urokinase-like plasminogen activator (UPA).

Plasmin digests fibrin (or fibrinogen) into fibrin degradation products (FDPs) and also degrades factors V and VII. Free plasmin is inactivated by plasma α_2-antiplasmin and α_2-macroglobulin.

Laboratory tests of coagulation

These are listed in Table 36.1.

Specialized tests

Individual coagulation factors can be assayed by functional tests or immunological methods. Platelet function tests include tests of platelet aggregation with different agonists; platelet function analyser-100 (PFA-100), which measures the length of time blood can be passed through a small orifice before the platelets completely occlude it; and platelet adhesion and assessment of platelet granule contents. Tests for abnormalities leading to thrombosis (thrombophilia) are described in Chapter 40.

37 Disorders of haemostasis I: vessel wall and platelets

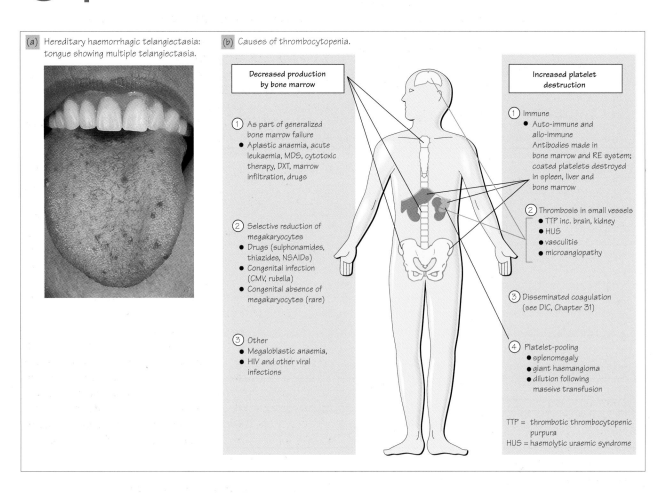

(a) Hereditary haemorrhagic telangiectasia: tongue showing multiple telangiectasia.

(b) Causes of thrombocytopenia.

Decreased production by bone marrow

① As part of generalized bone marrow failure
● Aplastic anaemia, acute leukaemia, MDS, cytotoxic therapy, DXT, marrow infiltration, drugs

② Selective reduction of megakaryocytes
● Drugs (sulphonamides, thiazides, NSAIDs)
● Congenital infection (CMV, rubella)
● Congenital absence of megakaryocytes (rare)

③ Other
● Megaloblastic anaemia,
● HIV and other viral infections

Increased platelet destruction

① Immune
● Auto-immune and allo-immune Antibodies made in bone marrow and RE system; coated platelets destroyed in spleen, liver and bone marrow

② Thrombosis in small vessels
● TTP inc. brain, kidney
● HUS
● vasculitis
● microangiopathy

③ Disseminated coagulation (see DIC, Chapter 31)

④ Platelet-pooling
● splenomegaly
● giant haemangioma
● dilution following massive transfusion

TTP = thrombotic thrombocytopenic purpura
HUS = haemolytic uraemic syndrome

Vessel wall abnormalities

These are associated with easy bruising, purpura and ecchymosis and spontaneous bleeding from mucosal surfaces. Tests of coagulation and platelet function are normal.

Inherited

• Hereditary haemorrhagic telangiectasia. This is autosomal dominant with multiple dilated microvascular swellings, typically in oropharynx (Fig. 37a) and gastrointestinal tract, which bleed spontaneously or following minor trauma. Local treatment (e.g. nasal packing) may control bleeding; tranexamic acid helps to reduce bleeding. Chronic iron deficiency is frequent.
• Ehlers–Danlos syndrome, Marfan's syndrome and other rare connective tissue disorders.

Acquired

Causes include vitamin C deficiency (scurvy), steroid therapy, normal ageing (senile purpura), amyloid in blood vessels and cryoglobulinaemia and immune complex deposition (e.g. pur-

pura fulminans in septicaemia). Henoch–Schönlein purpura is an allergic vasculitis which follows an acute infection, usually in childhood, and may be associated with arthropathy, haematuria and gastrointestinal symptoms.

Platelets

Excessive bleeding caused by thrombocytopenia or disordered platelet function is mucosal (e.g. epistaxis, gastrointestinal bleeding or menorrhagia) or affects the skin (purpura, petechiae and ecchymoses). Symptoms usually occur when the platelet count is $<10 \times 10^9$/L, but this may be higher when there is impaired platelet function. Thrombocytopenia (platelets $<140 \times 10^9$/L) (Fig. 37b) may be congenital or acquired. **Congenital** is rare; causes include congenital aplastic anaemia, thrombocytopenia with absent radii syndrome and Wiskott–Aldrich syndrome (thrombocytopenia with eczema and hypogammaglobulinaemia). Congenital infection (e.g. rubella, cytomegalovirus) frequently leads to thrombocytopenia. **Acquired** causes are deficient platelet production or accelerated platelet destruction.

Autoimmune thrombocytopenia

The platelets are coated with autoantibody (immunoglobulin) and are prematurely destroyed by the macrophages of the reticuloendothelial system. The acute form usually presents in childhood (2–7 years) and often follows a viral infection. Purpuric rash or epistaxis is frequent. It typically resolves spontaneously. A minority develop mucosal bleeding and should be treated with prednisolone or intravenous immunoglobulin. Up to 20% develop chronic immune thrombocytopenia.

Immune thrombocytopenia in adults is less likely to resolve without therapy and usually chronic. It is more common in females (M/F ratio is 1:4). Autoantibody is present on the platelet surface and may also be present as free antibody in serum.

Laboratory tests show normal haemoglobin and white cell count; low platelets (often $<20 \times 10^9/L$), normal bone marrow and normal coagulation. Immune thrombocytopenia also occurs in association with some malignancies (e.g. chronic lymphocytic leukaemia, non-Hodgkin lymphoma, myelodysplasia), infections (e.g. Epstein–Barr virus, HIV, malaria) and connective tissue disease (e.g. systemic lupus erythematosus). Patients should be tested for anti-nuclear factor (ANF) and anticardiolipin antibodies.

Treatment, if necessary, is with the following:
- Prednisolone (1 mg/kg/day, reducing over 4–6 weeks).
- Intravenous immunoglobulin is valuable for obtaining a temporary rise in platelet count.
- Splenectomy is required for non-responders with continuing symptoms and/or very low platelet counts.
- Additional immunosuppressive therapy (e.g. azathioprine, cyclophosphamide, cyclosporin A, rhesus anti-D, vincristine) or combination chemotherapy has been used. Rituximab (anti-CD20) and danazol are also of value in some cases.
- Synthetic activators of platelet function which function as thrombopoietin analogues are in clinical trial.

Alloimmune thrombocytopenia

Transplacental passage of maternal antibody in immune thrombocytopenia can lead to neonatal thrombocytopenia, which typically resolves spontaneously over a few weeks. Mothers who have been sensitized (e.g. by blood transfusion or previous pregnancy) to platelet antigens may develop antibodies which cross the placenta and coat foetal and neonatal platelets, which are then removed in the reticuloendothelial system. Individuals with such platelet alloantibodies can also become thrombocytopenic after blood transfusion (post-transfusion purpura). The antibody is then directed against the HPA1-a antigen on platelets.

Other causes of thrombocytopenia

Drugs cause thrombocytopenia by inhibiting marrow production or by an immune mechanism. The most common immune mechanism (e.g. quinine, heparin) is when the drug forms an antigen with a plasma protein, an antibody is formed to it, and circulating antigen–antibody complexes are absorbed on the platelet surface. Heparin-induced thrombocytopenia is associated with thrombosis. A 'heparinoid' drug is then used to continue anticoagulation.

Disseminated intravascular coagulation (Chapter 39)

Thrombotic thrombocytopenic purpura and haemolytic uraemic syndrome

Thrombotic thrombocytopenic purpura (**TTP**) and haemolytic uraemic syndrome (**HUS**) are characterized by thrombosis in small vessels, red cell fragmentation, haemolytic anaemia (see Fig. 17c) and thrombocytopenia. Fever, neurological changes and liver dysfunction occur in TTP and renal failure often occurs in HUS. The PT and APTT are normal.

TTP occurs in adults and may be associated with autoimmune conditions (e.g. SLE), pregnancy and infection. It is caused by a deficiency – either congenital or acquired due to an autoantibody – of a plasma protease ADAMTS-13 which normally cleaves von Willebrand factor (vWF). Abnormally high-molecular-weight vWF complexes are present in plasma. **HUS** occurs in childhood and follows infection with verotoxin-producing strains of *Escherichia coli*; or less frequently is associated with *Shigella*, *Salmonella* and streptococcal infection, pregnancy, autoimmune diseases and drugs (e.g. cyclosporin A). The ADAMTS-13 levels are normal.

Treatment of TTP is with plasma exchange using fresh frozen plasma (FFP) as the replacement fluid. Antiplatelet drugs (aspirin or dipyridamole), corticosteroids, splenectomy, rituximab and vincristine have all also been used. Response to treatment may be monitored by haemoglobin level, reticulocytes, lactate dehydrogenase, platelet count, plasma bilirubin and presence of vWF multimers in plasma. In HUS, treatment for fits, hypertension and renal failure are needed.

Disorders of platelet function (Table 37.1)

These are characterized by a prolonged bleeding time with normal platelet count, abnormal PFA-100 test and disordered platelet aggregation. **Inherited disorders** are rare and present with bruising/excessive bleeding after surgery or injury in childhood. The most common **acquired** cause is aspirin or other non-steroidal anti-inflammatory drugs.

Table 37.1 Disorders of platelet function (see Fig. 35b)

Inherited
 Bernard–Soulier syndrome (defective glycoprotein 1b, giant platelets)
 Glanzmann's thrombasthaenia (defective glycoproteins IIb, IIIa)
 Storage pool diseases, von Willebrand's disease

Acquired
 Drugs: aspirin, other non-steroidal anti-inflammatory agents, clopidogrel, dextran, antibiotics therapy (e.g. cephalosporins)
 Myeloproliferative disorders (see Chapters 26–28)
 Uraemia
 Paraproteinaemia, e.g. myeloma or Waldenström's macroglobulinaemia

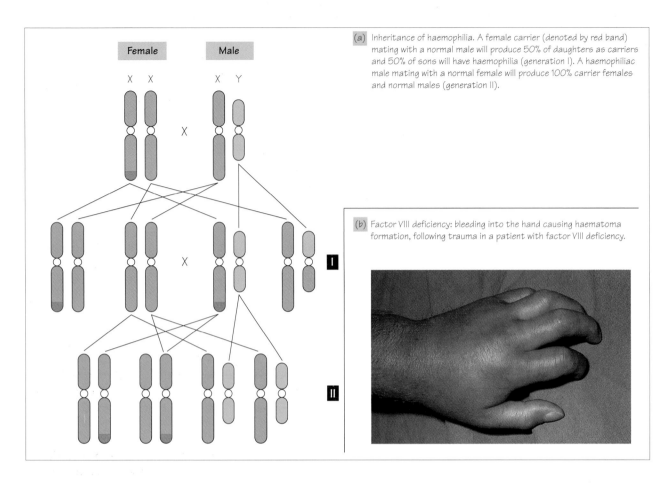

(a) Inheritance of haemophilia. A female carrier (denoted by red band) mating with a normal male will produce 50% of daughters as carriers and 50% of sons will have haemophilia (generation I). A haemophiliac male mating with a normal female will produce 100% carrier females and normal males (generation II).

(b) Factor VIII deficiency: bleeding into the hand causing haematoma formation, following trauma in a patient with factor VIII deficiency.

Excessive bleeding may occur as a result of an inherited defect of one or other protein involved in coagulation. Inherited deficiency of each of the coagulation factors is described.

Factor VIII deficiency (haemophilia A)

Factor VIII deficiency (haemophilia A) is the most common inherited coagulation disorder. The factor VIII gene is on the X chromosome so inheritance is sex-linked (Fig. 38a). A wide range of genetic changes including deletions, insertions, point mutations and a common intragene inversion underlie the disease.

Clinical features

- These range from severe spontaneous bleeding, especially into joints (haemarthroses) and muscles, to mild symptoms, depending on the factor VIII level (Fig. 38b).
- Onset in early childhood (e.g. postcircumcision).
- Increased risk of postoperative or post-traumatic haemorrhage.
- Chronic debilitating joint disease caused by repeated bleeds.
- Pseudotumours as a result of extensive fascial or subperiosteal bleeds.

Laboratory features (Table 38.1)

- Prolonged activated partial thromboplastin time (APTT), normal prothrombin time (PT), normal bleeding time, plasma factor VIII reduced (<1% of normal in severe cases, but up to 10% in mild cases).
- Carriers have factor VIII approximately 50% of normal. DNA analysis is helpful in carrier detection and antenatal diagnosis
- Von Willebrand factor (vWF) level is normal.

Treatment (see also Chapter 47)

- Infusions of factor VIII (either recombinant or concentrate from normal donated plasma) to elevate the patient's level to 20–50% of normal for severe bleeding.
- Level is raised to and maintained at 80–100% for elective surgery.
- Desmopressin, an analogue of vasopressin, leads to a modest rise in endogenous factor VIII which is useful in mild cases.
- Avoid aspirin, other antiplatelet drugs and intramuscular injections.
- Patients should be registered with a recognized haemophilia centre and should carry a card with details of their condition.
- Patients may need to have continuing or prophylactic treatment at home.

Table 38.1 Laboratory features of inherited coagulation disorders

Condition	PT	APTT	Bleeding time (or PFA-100)	Other
Haemophilia A	N	↑	N	Factor VIII ↓
Haemophilia B	N	↑	N	Factor IX ↓
von Willebrand's disease	N	↑	↑	von Willebrand factor ↓
				Factor VIII ↓
				Abnormal platelet aggregation with ristocetin

- Carrier detection and antenatal diagnosis can be carried out.
- Trials of gene therapy are under way.

Complications of treatment
• HIV and hepatitis C from impure preparations (prior to the early 1980s), subsequent AIDS, hepatitis and cirrhosis.
• Neutralizing antibodies to factor VIII in 15% of severe patients may require immunosuppressive therapy, treatment with porcine factor VIII, or plasma exchange.

Factor IX deficiency (haemophilia B, Christmas disease)
Factor IX deficiency (haemophilia B, Christmas disease) has similar clinical features to haemophilia A. Also sex-linked, it is four times less common and usually milder than haemophilia A. Diagnosis and treatment are similar to haemophilia A, except that factor IX concentrate is used for treatment and desmopressin is not effective.

von Willebrand's disease
von Willebrand's disease is usually autosomal dominant and results from mutations in the vWF gene. vWF is a large multimeric protein produced by endothelial cells, which carries factor VIII in plasma and mediates platelet adhesion to endothelium (see Chapter 35). The disease is more frequent than haemophilia A; males and females are affected equally.

Clinical features
• Bleeding, typically from mucous membranes (mouth, epistaxes, menorrhagia).
• Excess blood loss following trauma or surgery.
• Haemarthroses and muscle bleeding are rare.

Diagnosis
• APTT is prolonged, PT normal.
• Factor VIII and vWF levels are reduced.
• Bleeding time is prolonged.
• Defective platelet function, reduced aggregation with ristocetin.
• Mild thrombocytopenia may occur.
• The disease is divided into subtypes depending on whether there is a reduction in vWF or different types of functional defect.

Treatment
• Intermediate purity factor VIII concentrate (contains both vWF and factor VIII) for bleeding.
• Desmopressin is helpful for mild bleeding.
• Fibrinolytic inhibitors (e.g. tranexamic acid) are helpful.
• Carrier detection and antenatal diagnosis based on foetal DNA analysis is available.

Other conditions
Factor XI deficiency is less frequent than haemophilia A (higher incidence among Ashkenazi Jews) and is autosomal recessive. There is poor correlation between factor XI levels and symptoms. It is generally mild, but severe spontaneous and postsurgical bleeding may occur. Congenital deficiencies of factor II, V, VII, X and XIII are rare and usually cause mild bleeding disorders. Factor XII deficiency prolongs the APTT but does not cause clinical symptoms. Fibrinogen deficiency occurs as a moderately severe autosomal recessive disorder. Dysfibrinogenaemia (presence of a functionally abnormal molecule) is both a rare autosomal dominant disorder and a more common acquired disorder (liver disease, malignancy and systemic lupus erythematosus).

39 Disorders of haemostasis III: acquired disorders of coagulation

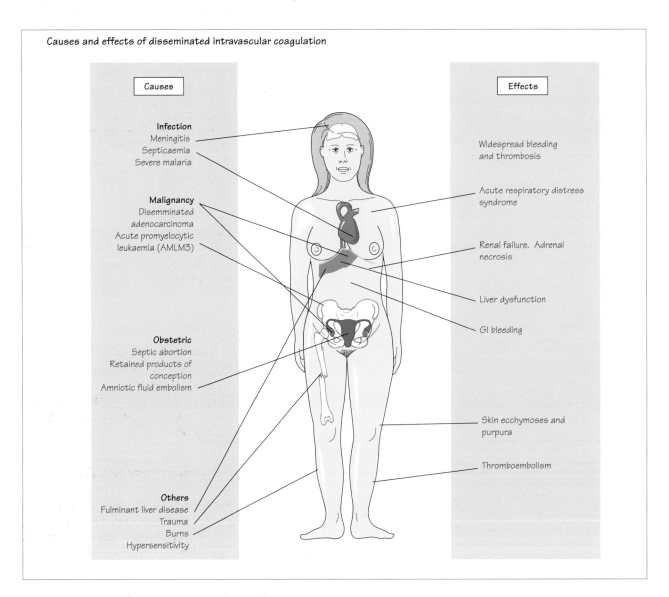

Causes and effects of disseminated intravascular coagulation

Causes

Infection
Meningitis
Septicaemia
Severe malaria

Malignancy
Disemminated
adenocarcinoma
Acute promyelocytic
leukaemia (AMLM3)

Obstetric
Septic abortion
Retained products of
conception
Amniotic fluid embolism

Others
Fulminant liver disease
Trauma
Burns
Hypersensitivity

Effects

Widespread bleeding
and thrombosis

Acute respiratory distress
syndrome

Renal failure. Adrenal
necrosis

Liver dysfunction

GI bleeding

Skin ecchymoses and
purpura

Thromboembolism

Liver disease

Liver disease leads to defects of coagulation, platelets and fibrinolysis.

• Reduced synthesis of vitamin K-dependent factors (II, VII, IX, X, proteins C and S) caused by impaired vitamin K absorption (biliary obstruction).

• Impaired synthesis of other coagulation proteins (factors I and V).

• Thrombocytopenia (hypersplenism) and abnormal platelet function (cirrhosis).

• Fibrinolysis impaired.

• Reduced levels of proteins C and S, antithrombin and α_2-antiplasmin lead to susceptibility to disseminated intravascular coagulation (DIC).

• Dysfibrinogenaemia may lead to haemorrhage or thrombosis.

Disseminated intravascular coagulation

Release of procoagulant material into the circulation or endothelial cell damage causes generalized activation of the coagulation and fibrinolytic pathways leading to widespread fibrin deposition in the circulation.

Clinical features

• Both bleeding and thrombosis may occur.

• Tissue damage caused by thrombosis leads to necrosis and further activation of coagulation and fibrinolysis.

• Purpura, ecchymoses, gastrointestinal bleeding, bleeding from intravenous sites and following venepuncture may occur as a result of low levels of coagulation factors and platelets resulting from increased consumption.

Table 39.1 Coagulation changes in acquired disorders of coagulation

	PT	APTT	TT	Platelets	Other
Liver disease	↑	↑	N/↑	↓	Dysfibrinogenaemia
DIC	↑	↑	↑	↓	FDP ↑ ± RBC fragments on blood film
Vitamin K deficiency	↑	↑ or N	N	N	
Massive transfusion	↑	↑	N	↓	
Oral anticoagulants	↑	↑	N	N	
Heparin	↑	↑	↑	N (rarely ↓)	Anti-Xa ↓

APTT, activated partial thromboplastin time; DIC, disseminated intravascular coagulation; FDP, fibrin degradation products; N, normal; PT, prothrombin time; RBC, red blood cell; TT, thrombin time

- Renal function may be impaired due to microvascular thrombosis.
- Other manifestations include acute respiratory distress syndrome (both a cause and a complication of DIC), adrenal necrosis, shock and thromboembolism.

Laboratory features (Table 39.1)
- Thrombocytopenia.
- Nearly all tests of coagulation and fibrinolysis are abnormal with low levels of fibrinogen.
- Fibrin degradation products (e.g. X-DP or FDP) are present in plasma (X = clotting factor).
- Blood film: microangiopathic haemolytic anaemia (see Fig. 17c) may occur.

Treatment
- Treat the cause, e.g. antibiotics, removal of the procoagulant stimulus (e.g. a dead foetus).
- Supportive therapy with fresh frozen plasma, platelet concentrates and cryoprecipitate if bleeding is dominant.
- Anticoagulant therapy (e.g. heparin) if thrombosis is dominant.
- Protein C concentrate and antithrombin in selected patients.

Other acquired disorders of coagulation
Drugs
- Anticoagulants and drugs affecting anticoagulation (see Chapter 41) are the most common drugs to disturb coagulation.
- Chemotherapy (e.g. L-asparaginase may lead to thrombosis).

Acquired coagulation inhibitors
These antibodies to coagulation factors are idiopathic, commoner in the elderly, or occur in malignancy (e.g. lymphoma), connective tissue disease (e.g. SLE) and with paraproteins (e.g. myeloma). They lead to excessive bleeding, both spontaneously and following injury.

Vitamin K deficiency
Vitamin K is required to activate factors II, VII, IX and X and protein C and S by γ-carboxylation (see Chapter 41). It is fat-soluble and derived from vegetables in food and intestinal flora. Deficiency occurs in patients on poor diets, those taking broad-spectrum antibiotics which reduce the gut flora, in biliary tract disease and with intestinal malabsorption.

Massive post-trauma/surgery uncontrollable bleeding
This can be due to multiple factors, DIC with consumption of platelets and clotting factors and excess fibrinolysis. If bleeding persists despite replacement of platelets and clotting factors, recombinant human factor VIIa may be life-saving.

Haemorrhagic disease of the newborn
Newborn infants are at an increased risk of bleeding because of hepatic immaturity and low levels of vitamin K. It is customary to give an injection of vitamin K (1 mg) to all newborn infants in the UK. Fears that this may lead to an increased risk of cancer have not been substantiated.

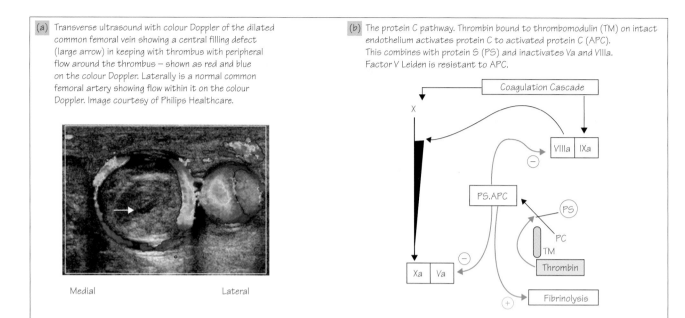

(a) Transverse ultrasound with colour Doppler of the dilated common femoral vein showing a central filling defect (large arrow) in keeping with thrombus with peripheral flow around the thrombus – shown as red and blue on the colour Doppler. Laterally is a normal common femoral artery showing flow within it on the colour Doppler. Image courtesy of Philips Healthcare.

Medial   Lateral

(b) The protein C pathway. Thrombin bound to thrombomodulin (TM) on intact endothelium activates protein C to activated protein C (APC). This combines with protein S (PS) and inactivates Va and VIIIa. Factor V Leiden is resistant to APC.

Thrombosis

Thrombosis is the pathological process whereby platelets and fibrin interact with the vessel wall to form a haemostatic plug to cause vascular obstruction. It may be arterial, causing ischaemia, or venous, leading to stasis (Fig. 40a). The thrombus may be subsequently lysed by fibrinolysis, organize, recanalize or embolize. Thrombosis underlies ischaemic heart, cerebrovascular and peripheral vascular disease; venous occlusion and pulmonary embolism; and it plays an important part in pre-eclampsia.

Arterial thrombosis

This occurs in relation to damaged endothelium, e.g. atherosclerotic plaques. Exposed collagen and released tissue factor cause platelet aggregation and fibrin formation (Table 40.1).

Venous thrombosis

Factors affecting blood flow (e.g. stasis, obesity), alterations in blood constituents and damage to vascular endothelium (e.g. caused by sepsis, surgery or indwelling catheters) are important risk factors. Diagnosis can be confirmed by imaging, e.g. venography or more commonly by Doppler ultrasound probe (Fig. 40a). Blood tests, e.g. detection of elevated levels of D-dimers, which are derived from fibrinogen, can also be helpful, especially if recurrence is suspected (Table 40.2).

Thrombophilia

Thrombophilia is a congenital or acquired predisposition to thrombosis. It should be suspected and screened for in patients with thrombosis who are young, have a positive family history, thrombosis in an unusual site or recurrence, and in females with recurrent foetal loss.

Inherited thrombophilia

This has been increasingly recognized recently (Tables 40.1 and 40.2; Fig. 40b). Presentation may be during early childhood or in adulthood, e.g. at commencement of oral contraceptives or during pregnancy/puerperium, after surgery or after a long haul flight. Inheritance of a variant form of factor V (factor V Leiden) is the most common (up to 5% of the population). Activated factor V Leiden is relatively resistant to inactivation by protein C. The risk of thrombosis is increased 5- to 10-fold in heterozygotes, and 50- to 100-fold in homozygotes. Rarer causes include protein C, protein S or antithrombin deficiency or functional abnormality, defective fibrinolysis (e.g. TPAI deficiency, see Chapter 36), mutant prothrombin and homocystinuria. The combination of two abnormalities often underlies severe cases.

Acquired thrombophilia

Acquired hypercoagulable states are listed in Tables 40.1 and 40.2. Pathogenesis, e.g. in pregnancy, oral contraceptive pill therapy and malignancy, is multifactorial and relates to elevated levels of procoagulant factors, depressed levels of inhibitor proteins and physical factors (e.g. stasis, surgery).

Lupus anticoagulant syndrome

Despite its name, this syndrome usually presents with arterial or venous thrombosis or recurrent miscarriages. It may be associated with systemic lupus erythematosus or other connective tissue disorders, with malignancy or infections or may be idiopathic. Patients may show a spectrum of antibodies which interfere with phospholipid-dependent coagulation tests in vitro and/or react with cardiolipin. The activated partial thromboplastin time is prolonged and not corrected by a 50:50 mix of normal plasma in patient plasma. Anticoagulant therapy is needed for patients with thrombosis.

Antiplatelet therapy

The use of heparin and warfarin is discussed in Chapter 41. Antiplatelet drugs (see Chapter 00) and fibrinolytic drugs are discussed here.

- Aspirin (75 mg daily and 300 mg post-myocardial infarction) is most widely used. It inhibits platelet function by inhibiting cyclo-oxygenase, thus reducing thromboxane A_2 production.
- Others: clopidogrel and monoclonal antibodies directed to platelet glycoproteins (e.g. abciximab, which is directed against glycoprotein IIb/IIIa) or small molecule inhibitors of glyco-protein IIb/IIIa eptifibatide or tirofiban are used, for example, post-angioplasty or stent insertion. The combination of aspirin and clopidogrel is used in high-risk cases and for the first year after angioplasty and stent insertion.

Indications

Prevention of thrombosis in patients with
- previous myocardial infarction, transient ischaemic attacks and stroke or high risk of first myocardial infarct in males;
- thrombocytosis, e.g. myeloproliferative disorders, post-splenectomy;
- prosthetic valves and post-coronary artery surgery or angio-plasty;
- pre-eclampsia and
- severe peripheral vascular disease.

Fibrinolytic therapy

This is used to enhance conversion of plasminogen to plasmin (see Chapter 36), which degrades fibrin. It must be used within 5–7 days for venous thrombi and 5–7 hours for arterial thrombi.
- Streptokinase directly activates plasminogen. Most individuals have antistreptococcal antibodies; a loading dose is therefore required and treatment becomes ineffective after 4–10 days.
- Urokinase has a similar action but may be used if there are high levels of antistreptococcal antibodies. Single-chain urokinase-type plasminogen activator (SCU-PA) has also been developed.
- Acylated plasminogen streptokinase activator complex (AP-SAC) activates streptokinase bound to plasminogen.
- Recombinant tissue plasminogen activation (TPA) causes activation of fibrin-bound plasminogen only, and is associated with less systemic activation of fibrinolysis.

Indications

- Acute myocardial infarction: streptokinase is usually given with 300 mg aspirin and heparin intravenously.
- Treatment of arterial and venous thrombosis, e.g. pulmonary embolism, peripheral arterial or venous thrombosis.
- In selected patients with acute stroke, after CT scan has confirmed absence of haemorrhage.

Table 40.1 Risk factors for arterial thrombosis

Hypertension

Smoking

Diabetes*

Hyperlipidaemia*

↑Homocysteine*

Polycythaemia/thrombocythaemia

↑Factor VIII

↑Fibrinogen

Lupus anticoagulant

*May be related to an inherited abnormality

Table 40.2 Risk factors for venous thrombosis

Conditions causing stasis
   Cardiac failure, oedema, nephrotic syndrome
   Postoperative
   Immobility and bed rest
   Trauma
   Pelvic obstruction
Altered blood constituents
   Coagulation factors
      Hereditary
         Factor V Leiden
         Protein C deficiency
         Protein S deficiency
         Antithrombin deficiency
         Prothrombin mutation
      Acquired
         Oestrogen therapy, contraceptive pill
         Malignancy
         Pregnancy and puerperium
         Lupus anticoagulant
         Raised plasma homocysteine (may also be inherited)
   Blood cells
      Polycythaemia
      Thrombocythaemia

Contraindications

- Patients with active gastrointestinal bleeding, aortic dissection, head injury or recent (<2 mo) neurosurgery, and bleeding diathesis.

Side effects

- Bleeding, especially in patients taking anticoagulants or antiplatelet drugs.
- Anaphylactic reactions may occur with streptokinase.

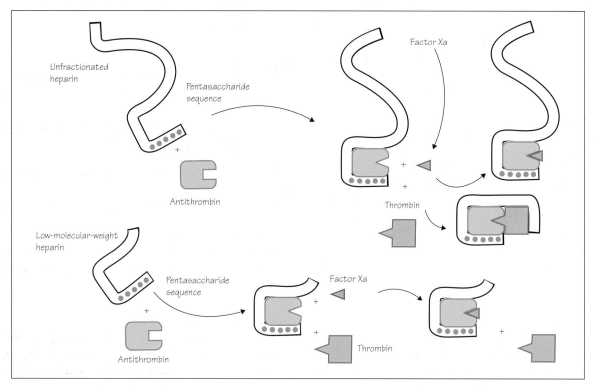

(a) Heparin binds to antithrombin via a pentasaccharide sequence and induces a conformational change which allows antithrombin to bind Xa and thrombin. The shorter chain length of low-molecular-weight heparin allows binding to only Xa, while unfractionated heparin will bind both Xa and thrombin. Thus, LMW heparin allows a selective inhibition of factor Xa. Modified from Weitz J.I. (1997) Low molecular-weight heparin. *New England Journal of Medicine*, **337**: 688–98.

(b) Action of warfarin.

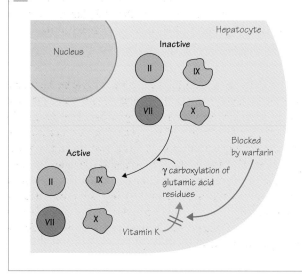

Unfractionated heparin (UFH) is a heterogeneous mixture of polysaccharide chains. Low-molecular-weight (LMW) heparin preparations (MW < 5000) have a greater ability to inactivate Xa and less effect on thrombin (Fig. 41a) and platelet function, and therefore have a lesser tendency to cause bleeding. They have a longer plasma half-life so that once daily subcutaneous administration is effective in prophylaxis. They also interact less than UFH with endothelium, plasma proteins, macrophages and platelets, making their action more predictable and eliminating the need for monitoring except in certain individuals (see below).

Indications

• Acute venous thrombosis, e.g. deep vein thrombosis (DVT) and pulmonary embolism. Continuous intravenous infusion of UFH for 5–7 days until warfarinized. Subcutaneous LMW heparin at a therapeutic dose is equally effective. Warfarin is usually started 1–2 days after heparin and heparin discontinued when international normalized ratio (INR) (see below) is >2.0.

• Unstable angina, post-myocardial infarction.

• Disseminated intravascular coagulation if this is dominated by thrombosis.

• Acute peripheral arterial occlusion.

Heparin

Heparin is a mucopolysaccharide which is not absorbed when given orally and is therefore given subcutaneously or intravenously. It activates antithrombin which irreversibly inactivates prothrombin, Xa, IXa and XIa. It also impairs platelet function.

- Prophylaxis of DVT in surgical patients (LMW heparin once daily).
- Thrombosis prophylaxis in patients undergoing cardiac surgery or renal dialysis.
- Pregnancy. As warfarin is teratogenic, heparin is used in pregnancy when anticoagulation is needed.
- Recurrent foetal loss.
- Maintaining patency of indwelling lines and catheters.

Monitoring

For continuous intravenous infusion, the APTT should be maintained at 1.5–2 × normal. LMW heparin therapy is not normally monitored; if necessary, e.g. in renal failure or in those of very low (<50 kg) or high (>80 kg) body weight, by factor Xa assay.

Side effects

- Haemorrhage, particularly if combined with antiplatelet therapy, overdosage or, rarely, platelet function defect. Heparin has a short half-life (1 h); levels fall rapidly when infusion stopped. Protamine sulphate will reverse heparin immediately but must be used with caution as it can cause haemorrhage at high dosage.
- Long-term therapy (>2 mo) can lead to osteoporosis.
- Thrombocytopenia, which is antibody-mediated. Platelet clumping may cause arterial thrombosis.
- LMW heparin is less likely than UFH to cause all these side effects.

Warfarin

Vitamin K promotes the γ-carboxylation of glutamic acid residues of factor II, VII, IX and X; warfarin prevents this to cause a 50% drop of factor VII levels within 24 hours and of factor II in 4 days. Full anticoagulation occurs 48–72 hours after starting warfarin therapy. Non-carboxylated factors II, VII, IX and X (proteins formed in vitamin K absence, PIVKAs) appear in plasma (see Fig. 41b). Protein C and S levels also fall and this initially (first 2–3 days) leads to an increased risk of thrombosis and may lead to skin necrosis, in those with protein C or S deficiency.

The therapeutic dose of warfarin is very variable, ranging from 0.5 to 20 mg daily. This depends largely on individual variation in its metabolism.

Control of therapy

The prothrombin time is measured and expressed as an INR against the mean normal prothrombin time using a calibrated thromboplastin. Treatment is monitored by maintaining the INR at 2.0–3.0 for most indications, but 2.5–3.5 for those with mechanical heart values and others at particular risk of thrombosis.

Indications

- Treatment of DVT, pulmonary embolism, systemic embolism (3–6-mo therapy).
- Prophylaxis against thrombosis in patients with atrial fibrillation, prosthetic valves, arterial grafts, repeated pulmonary embolism and in patients with two or more previous (especially if spontaneous) DVT.
- Low doses (to maintain INR 1.5) of value in prevention of myocardial infarct in high-risk groups.

Side effects

- Haemorrhage – especially in patients taking other anticoagulants, antiplatelet drugs or thrombolytic therapy, and in those with liver disease.

Drug interactions

Warfarin is tightly bound to albumin and is metabolized by the liver. The minor unbound fraction is active. Action is increased by drugs which
- reduce its binding to albumin, e.g. aspirin, sulphonamides;
- inhibit hepatic metabolism, e.g. allopurinol, tricyclic antidepressants, sulphonamides;
- decrease absorption of vitamin K, e.g. antibiotics, laxatives and
- decrease synthesis of vitamin K factors, e.g. high-dose salicylates.

Action is decreased by drugs which
- accelerate its metabolism, e.g. barbiturates, rifampicin and
- enhance synthesis of coagulation factors, e.g. oral contraceptives, hormone replacement therapy.

Reversal of action

Patients with haemorrhage and a raised INR should receive fresh frozen plasma or prothombin concentrates (of factors II, VII, IX and X). If severe, also vitamin K (10 mg intravenous) could be taken, but this results in resistance to warfarin for 2–3 weeks. Raised INR without haemorrhage is managed by withholding therapy for 1–2 days and repeating the INR, but if other risk factors exist, vitamin K, 1–2 mg orally, should be given.

Other anticoagulant drugs

The identification of thrombin receptors has led to development of receptor antagonist drugs. Hirudin, available as recombinant products lepirudin, bivalirudin and argatroban, is a specific direct inhibitor of thrombin. The preparations are licensed for intravenous use in adults who cannot receive heparin (e.g. because of heparin-induced thrombocytopenia) and are also used in coronary angioplasty and stenting. Fondaparinux is a direct inhibitor of factor X used parenterally in prophylaxis of DVT in orthopaedic patients. Orally active direct thrombin or Xa inhibitors are in trial and may well replace warfarin as they do not require patient monitoring.

Other treatments

Graduated elastic compression stockings help to prevent DVT post-operatively and to prevent a post-phlebitis syndrome occurring after DVT. An inferior vena cava filter may be inserted to reduce the risk of pulmonary embolus in selected cases.

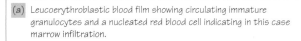

(a) Leucoerythroblastic blood film showing circulating immature granulocytes and a nucleated red blood cell indicating in this case marrow infiltration.

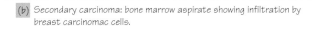

(b) Secondary carcinoma: bone marrow aspirate showing infiltration by breast carcinomac cells.

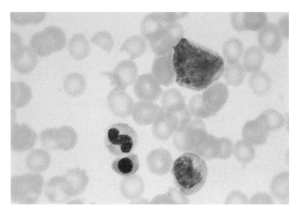

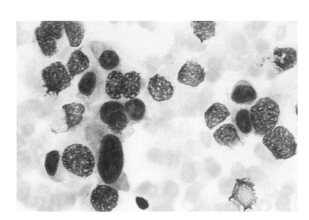

(c) Secondary carcinoma: bone marrow aspirate immunocytochemistry showing positive staining for cytokeratin in breast carcinoma cells.

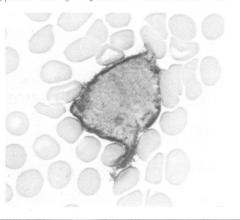

A wide range of abnormalities affecting red cells, white cells, platelets and coagulation factors occur in association with systemic illness.

Anaemia of chronic disease

- Anaemia of chronic disease (ACD) is a common normochromic or mildly hypochromic anaemia, occurring in patients with a systemic disease (Table 42.1).
- Moderate anaemia occurs, haemoglobin level > 9.0 g/dL, severity of anaemia correlating with severity of underlying disease.
- Reduced serum iron and total iron-binding capacity.
- Normal or raised serum ferritin with adequate iron stores in the bone marrow but stainable iron absent from erythroblasts.
- Usually the erythrocyte sedimentation rate and C-reactive protein are raised.

Pathogenesis

Hepcidin, released by the liver in response to inflammatory cytokines, reduces iron absorption and iron release by macrophages into plasma. Increased levels of cytokines, especially IL-1, IL-6, tumour necrosis factor and interferon-γ, interact with accessory marrow stromal cells, macrophages and erythroid progenitors to reduce erythropoiesis, iron utilization and response to erythropoietin (EPO).

Treatment

- Therapy of the chronic disease gradually reduces levels of mediator cytokines.
- Recombinant EPO may improve anaemia in patients with, e.g. rheumatoid arthritis (RA), cancer and myeloma.

Table 42.1 Conditions associated with anaemia of chronic disease

Chronic infections
Especially osteomyelitis, bacterial endocarditis, tuberculosis, chronic abscesses, bronchiectasis, chronic urinary tract infections, HIV, AIDS, malaria

Other chronic inflammatory disorders
Rheumatoid arthritis, polymyalgia rheumatica, systemic lupus erythematosus, scleroderma, inflammatory bowel disease, thrombophlebitis

Malignant diseases
Carcinoma, especially metastatic or associated with infection, lymphoma

Others
Congestive heart failure, ischaemic heart disease

Malignancy

Anaemia

- ACD affects almost all cancer patients at some stage.
- Blood loss in gastrointestinal and gynaecological malignancies.
- Autoimmune haemolytic anaemia, especially in lymphoma.
- Microangiopathic haemolytic anaemia (see Chapter 17) may occur with disseminated mucin-secreting adenocarcinoma.
- Leucoerythroblastic anaemia indicates marrow infiltration by tumour (Fig. 41a).
- Red cell aplasia is associated with thymoma, lymphoma and chronic lymphocytic leukaemia.
- Chemotherapy or radiotherapy-induced inhibition of bone marrow.
- Folate deficiency as a result of poor diet and widespread disease.

Polycythaemia

Tumour cells may produce EPO or EPO-like peptides in renal cell carcinoma, hepatoma and uterine myoma (see Chapter 26).

White cell changes

Cancer patients frequently have opportunistic infections or bleed, which raises white cells (usually neutrophils), or receive chemotherapy or radiotherapy, which lowers them.

Platelets

Thrombocytopenia may be due to decreased production, e.g. extensive marrow infiltration, chemotherapy or radiotherapy, accelerated peripheral destruction, e.g. disseminated intravascular coagulation (DIC) and/or hypersplenism (Fig. 37c). Immune thrombocytopenia may occur especially with lymphoma.

Thrombocytosis is a frequent reactive phenomenon in malignancy (see Chapter 26).

Coagulation changes

Activation of both coagulation and fibrinolysis may predispose to either haemorrhage or thrombosis. Chronic DIC, e.g. with pancreatic carcinoma, causes thrombosis, including migratory thrombophlebitis (Trousseau's syndrome). Circulating anticoagulants, e.g. acquired von Willebrand factor inhibitors, and specific coagulation factor inhibitors may occur.

Connective tissue disorders

Anaemia

- ACD is common. Iron deficiency may coexist in patients with gastrointestinal haemorrhage caused by non-steroidal anti-inflammatory agents.
- Autoimmune haemolytic anaemia occurs in systemic lupus erythematosus (SLE), RA and mixed connective tissue disorders.
- Red cell aplasia occurs in SLE.

White cells

Inflammation leads to neutrophilia. Neutropenia with splenomegaly occurs in patients with RA (Felty's syndrome). Antibody and immune complex-mediated neutrophil destruction and decreased neutrophil production in the marrow may also occur in SLE. Eosinophilia may occur in SLE, RA and polyarteritis nodosa.

Platelets

Thrombocytopenia may be immune (SLE and RA). Thrombocytosis is a non-specific reactive phenomenon to inflammation in connective tissue disorders.

Coagulation changes

These may be caused by associated renal disease, drug therapy, DIC and specific coagulation factor inhibitors. The lupus anticoagulant occurs in approximately 10% of patients with SLE (see Chapter 40).

43

Haematological aspects of systemic disease II: renal, liver, endocrine, amyloid

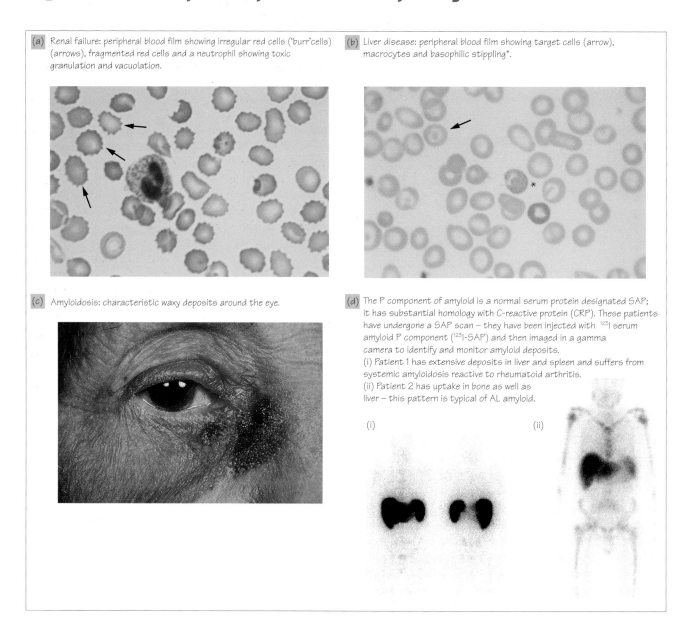

(a) Renal failure: peripheral blood film showing irregular red cells ('burr'cells) (arrows), fragmented red cells and a neutrophil showing toxic granulation and vacuolation.

(b) Liver disease: peripheral blood film showing target cells (arrow), macrocytes and basophilic stippling*.

(c) Amyloidosis: characteristic waxy deposits around the eye.

(d) The P component of amyloid is a normal serum protein designated SAP; it has substantial homology with C-reactive protein (CRP). These patients have undergone a SAP scan – they have been injected with ^{123}I serum amyloid P component (^{123}I-SAP) and then imaged in a gamma camera to identify and monitor amyloid deposits.
(i) Patient 1 has extensive deposits in liver and spleen and suffers from systemic amyloidosis reactive to rheumatoid arthritis.
(ii) Patient 2 has uptake in bone as well as liver – this pattern is typical of AL amyloid.

(i)   (ii)

Renal disease
Anaemia

Acute or chronic renal failure causes a normochromic, normocytic anaemia, with reduced erythropoietin (EPO) levels – the main cause of anaemia – and echinocytes (burr cells) in the blood film (Fig. 43a). Iron deficiency (blood loss) and haemolysis in haemolytic uraemic syndrome and thrombotic thrombocytopenic purpura are other causes. EPO corrects anaemia up to a haemoglobin level of 12 g/dL. A poor response to EPO occurs with iron or folate deficiency, haemolysis, infection, occult malignancy, aluminium toxicity, hyperparathyroidism and inadequate dialysis. Hypertension and thrombosis of an arteriovenous fistula may occur with EPO therapy.

Polycythaemia

Polycythaemia may occur with renal tumours or cysts.

Haemostatic abnormalities

Coagulation factors II, XI or XIII may be reduced and platelet function is impaired (predispose to bleeding), whereas low levels of protein C, AT or plasminogen may lead to thrombosis.

Endocrine disease
Anaemia

Both hyper- and hypothyroidism cause mild anaemia (mean corpuscular volume raised in hypothyroidism, low in thyrotoxicosis). Deficiencies of iron, as a result of menorrhagia or achlorhydria, or B_{12} (increased incidence of pernicious anaemia in hypothyroidism, hypoadrenalism and hypoparathyroidism), may complicate the anaemia. Antithyroid drugs (carbimazole and propylthiouracil) can cause aplastic anaemia or agranulocytosis.

Liver disease
Anaemia
This may be caused by anaemia of chronic disease, haemodilution (increased plasma volume), pooling of red cells (splenomegaly) and haemorrhage, e.g. caused by oesophageal varices. The mean corpuscular volume is raised, particularly in alcoholics, and target cells, echinocytes and acanthocytes, occur in the blood film (Fig. 43b). Haemolysis and hypertriglyceridaemia with alcoholic liver disease (Zieve's syndrome) is rare. Direct toxicity of copper for red cells causes haemolysis in Wilson's disease. Viral hepatitis, including hepatitis A, B and C and hepatitis viruses yet to be characterized, may lead to aplastic anaemia.

Platelets and haemostasis
Platelets may be low (hypersplenism or disseminated intravascular coagulation). Coagulation abnormalities are discussed in Chapter 39.

Amyloid
Amyloidosis is the tissue deposition of a fibrillary homogeneous eosinophilic protein material which is birefringent and stains with Congo red. It is classified into

• amyloid derived from clonal lymphocyte or plasma cell proliferation (AL) (e.g. myeloma, primary amyloidosis) when immunoglobulin light chains or components of them are deposited (see Chapter 30) and
• reactive amyloidosis (AA) which occurs when serum amyloid A protein, an apolipoprotein, is deposited as a result of a chronic inflammatory disease, e.g. rheumatoid arthritis, inflammatory bowel disease or chronic infection, e.g. tuberculosis, leprosy, osteomyelitis and bronchiectasis. Familial Mediterranean fever is a chronic inflammatory disease often affecting the kidneys and joints in which amyloidosis is a frequent complication. It is due to mutation of the pyrinin gene. The protein affects complement activation and neutrophil function.

Localized amyloid occurs in, for example, endocrine organs or skin in old age (Fig. 43c), with deposition of protein A, hormones and other constituents. There are also a number of rare inherited forms of amyloid due to genetic abnormalities in various proteins.

Amyloid P protein is a serum protein related to C-reactive protein, which is deposited in both AL and AA types of amyloid. Amyloid deposition leads to organ enlargement and dysfunction. Tissues involved include kidneys, heart, skin, tongue, endocrine organs, liver, spleen, gastrointestinal and respiratory tracts and the autonomic nervous system. Diagnosis is made by biopsy of tongue, gums, abdominal fat or rectum with special staining. The extent of the disease can be measured using radioactive-labelled P-protein and whole-body scanning (Fig. 43d).

Haematological aspects of systemic disease III: infection

(a) Haemophagocytic syndrome: bone marrow aspirate showing a macrophage laden with cellular debris.

(b) Malaria: peripheral blood film showing red cells invaded by ring forms of *Plasmodium falciparum*.

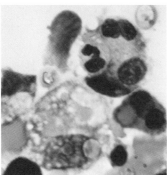

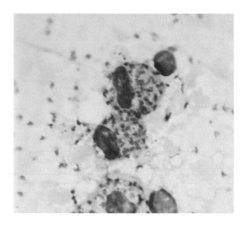

(c) Malaria life cycle. 1, Sporozoites, injected through the skin by female anopheline mosquito; 2, sporozoites infect hepatocytes; 3, some sporozoites develop into 'hypnozoites' (*Plasmodium vivax* and *P. ovale* only); 4, liver-stage parasite develops; 5–6, tissue schizogony; 7, merozoites are released into the circulation; 8, ring-stage trophozoites in red cells; 9, erythrocytic schizogony; 10, merozoites invade other red cells; 11, some parasites develop into female (macro-) or male (micro gametocytes, taken up by mosquito; 12, mature macrogametocyte and exflagellating microgametes; 13, ookinete penetrates gut wall; 14, development of oocyst; 15, sporozoites penetrate salivary glands.

(d) Leishmaniasis: bone marrow aspirate showing a macrophage containing Leishman–Donovan bodies.

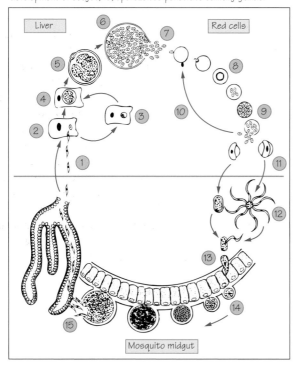

Haematology at a Glance, 3e. By A. Mehta and V. Hoffbrand. Published 2009 by Blackwell Publishing. ISBN 978-1-4051-7970-6.

Infections

Viruses

Anaemia

Autoimmune haemolytic anaemia may occur, especially, in infectious mononucleosis, usually of cold type. B_{19} parvovirus causes erythema variegata or fifth disease in children and leads to transient red cell aplasia in patients with haemolytic anaemia (aplastic crisis). Anaemia occurs with pancytopenia in virus-associated bone marrow aplasia (hepatitis viruses, HIV and cytomegalovirus in organ transplant recipients). Microangiopathic haemolytic anaemia (MAHA) with thrombotic thrombocytopenic purpura (TTP) may occur with various viral infections.

White cells

Typically neutropenia with lymphopenia or lymphocytosis (see Chapter 9) occurs.

Platelets

Thrombocytopenia may be immune (e.g. infectious mononucleosis, HIV) caused by bone marrow aplasia, or by increased consumption – disseminated intravascular coagulation (DIC), haemophagocytosis (Fig. 44a), haemolytic uraemic syndrome and TTP. Reactive thrombocytosis can also occur.

Bacterial, fungal and protozoal infection

Anaemia

Anaemia of chronic disease is frequent. Haemolytic anaemia may be immune (e.g. cold antibodies with anti-I specificity in mycoplasma infection) or non-immune (e.g. direct red cell invasion, *Bartonella bacilliformis*; or toxin-mediated, *Clostridium perfringens* and *Staphylococcus aureus*). DIC and MAHA may occur. Haemolytic uraemic syndrome may follow infection by verotoxin-producing strains of *Escherichia coli*, *Salmonella*, *Shigella* and *Campylobacter*. Blood loss can occur with *Helicobacter pylori* and ankylostoma infections.

White cells

Neutrophilia is most common (see Chapter 9).

Platelets

Thrombocytosis is frequently reactive. Thrombocytopenia may also occur, caused by immune destruction, circulating immune complexes, decreased platelet production and DIC in severe bacterial, fungal and rickettsial infection.

Haemostasis

DIC may dominate the clinical picture in certain infections, e.g. bacterial meningitis.

Malaria (Figs. 44b and 44c)

Anaemia is caused by haemolysis (cellular disruption and haemoglobin digestion), splenic sequestration, haemodilution (raised plasma volume) and ineffective erythropoiesis. Malarial antigens attached to red cells may cause immune haemolysis. Acute intravascular haemolysis with haemoglobinuria and renal failure (blackwater fever) occurs rarely in *Plasmodium falciparum* infection. Anaemia of chronic disease may also occur. Eosinophilia is variable. Thrombocytopenia (in up to 70% of *P. falciparum* infections) may be caused by immune destruction, splenic sequestration and DIC.

Leishmaniasis

Visceral leishmaniasis is a protozoal infection caused by *Leishmania donovani*. Hepatosplenomegaly, hypergammaglobulinaemia, normochromic anaemia and a raised ESR occur. Bone marrow aspirate shows macrophages containing Leishman–Donovan bodies (Fig. 44d).

HIV infection and AIDS

HIV-1 is a retrovirus transmitted by semen, blood and other body fluids, which infects and kills $CD4^+$ T lymphocytes to cause immune suppression. A non-specific febrile illness with lymphadenopathy often marks initial infection. A proportion of patients progress to AIDS with a CD4 count $<0.2 \times 10^9$/L. Clinical manifestations include recurring infections, anaemia and lymphadenopathy. There is an increased risk of non-Hodgkin lymphoma (especially high grade and involving the CNS), Kaposi's sarcoma and other tumours, e.g. Hodgkin's disease, acute myeloid leukaemia. Treatment may also induce anaemia; e.g. both azidothymidine (AZT) and co-trimoxazole cause megaloblastic change. Thrombocytopenia, lymphopenia and neutropenia (immune or caused by marrow failure or drug therapy) are also frequent. The bone marrow is usually normo- or hypercellular, with dysplastic features and an increase in plasma cells. A serum paraprotein occurs in 10–15% of cases.

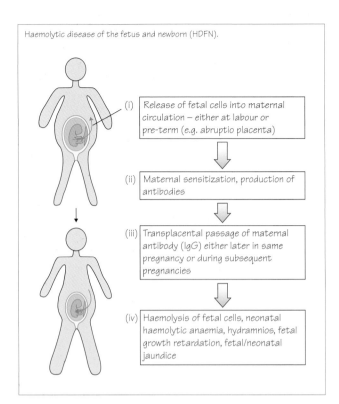

Haemolytic disease of the fetus and newborn (HDFN).

(i) Release of fetal cells into maternal circulation – either at labour or pre-term (e.g. abruptio placenta)

(ii) Maternal sensitization, production of antibodies

(iii) Transplacental passage of maternal antibody (IgG) either later in same pregnancy or during subsequent pregnancies

(iv) Haemolysis of fetal cells, neonatal haemolytic anaemia, hydramnios, fetal growth retardation, fetal/neonatal jaundice

Anaemia

Plasma volume increases by up to 50% during first and second trimesters, whereas red cell mass (RCM) increases by only 20–30%. Haemodilution results (haemoglobin falls to a mean 10.5 g/dL between 16 and 40 weeks). A physiological rise in mean corpuscular volume of 5–10 fl occurs. Increase in RCM, iron transfer to the foetus and blood loss during labour together require about 1000 mg of iron, so that iron deficiency is frequent. Folate requirements rise because of increased catabolism. Early supplementation (e.g. 400 μg daily) reduces risk of megaloblastic anaemia and of foetal neural tube defects (see Chapter 14). The serum B_{12} level falls below normal in 20–30% of pregnant woman, to rise again spontaneously post-delivery. Autoimmune haemolytic anaemia in pregnancy is typically severe and refractory to therapy. Haemolytic anaemia with elevated liver enzymes and low platelets (HELLP syndrome) and epigastric pain may occur in the last trimester. Disseminated intravascular coagulation (DIC) may accompany HELLP syndrome and induction of labour or caesarean section is often necessary.

White cells

Mild neutrophil leucocytosis with a left shift.

Platelets

Gestational thrombocytopenia complicates 8–10% of pregnancies, is mild (platelets $80–150 \times 10^9$/L) and is not associated with neonatal thrombocytopenia or significant bleeding. Maternal immune thrombocytopenic purpura may antedate or present in pregnancy and is associated with increased levels of platelet-associated IgG or serum platelet autoantibodies. Management includes no therapy (absence of bleeding, platelets $>50 \times 10^9$/L), corticosteroids or intravenous immunoglobulin, which also crosses placenta to elevate the foetal platelet count. Thrombocytopenia occurs in pre-eclampsia (mechanism unknown); low-dose aspirin therapy may reduce platelet consumption.

Coagulation changes

Coagulation changes (Table 45.1) combine to give an increased risk of thrombosis and DIC. This occurs in up to 40% of cases of abruptio placenta, leading to haemorrhage and shock. Retention of a dead foetus usually leads to chronic low-grade DIC with onset over 1–2 weeks. Venous stasis resulting from the gravid uterus combines with these changes to make pregnancy a hypercoagulable state; operative delivery imposes an additional risk of pastpartum DVT.

Haemolytic disease of the foetus and newborn

Haemolytic disease of the foetus and newborn (HDFN) is the haemolysis of foetal or neonatal red cells caused by transplacental passage of maternal red cell antibodies (see figure).

HDFN caused by ABO antibodies

Although ABO incompatibility between mother and foetus is common, this type of HDFN is rarely severe. Most ABO antibodies are IgM and therefore cannot cross the placenta. Foetal A and B antigens are not fully developed at birth, and the maternal antibodies can be partially neutralized by A and B antigens present on other cells, in the plasma and in the tissue fluids.

HDFN caused by Rh and other antibodies

The most important cause is anti-D, produced in Rh(D)-negative woman as a result of sensitization during a previous miscarriage, pregnancy or blood transfusion and causing haemolysis in Rh(D)-positive infants. Other important causes are other antibodies with the Rh system, e.g. anti-C. Anti-Kell, anti-Duffy and anti-JKa antibodies may also rarely cause HDFN.

Haemolysis of foetal cells can lead to hydrops foetalis, though nowadays it more commonly leads to neonatal haemolytic anaemia. All women must have their blood group determined at booking and atypical red cell antibodies in plasma should be detected. If present, their titre is monitored throughout pregnancy. Ultrasound for foetal growth, foetal blood sampling and measurements of bilirubin levels in amniotic fluid are used to monitor foetal well-being.

Treatment

Foetuses may be given transfusion of fresh red cells (CMV negative, irradiated) compatible with maternal serum. Maternal antibody levels can be lowered by plasma exchange.

Table 45.1 Haemostatic changes during pregnancy

Coagulation factors
   Vitamin K-dependent factors II, VII, IX, X ↑
   Factor VII ↑, von Willebrand factor ↑
   Fibrinogen ↑

Coagulation inhibitors
   Protein C ↑ or no change
   Antithrombin ↑ or no change

Fibrinolytic activity
   Reduced

Thrombocytopenia
   Gestational
   Immune
   Pre-eclampsia
   Thrombotic thrombocytopenic purpura (typically mid-trimester)
   Haemolytic uraemic syndrome (typically post-delivery)
   HELLP syndrome

HELLP, haemolytic anaemia with elevated liver enzymes and low platelets

Phototherapy and exchange transfusion of the neonate allow removal of unconjugated bilirubin, which may otherwise deposit in the basal ganglia to cause neurological sequelae (kernicterus).

Prevention

This is by administration of anti-D to unsensitized Rh(D)-negative women within 72 hours of a potentially sensitizing event (e.g. birth of an Rh(D)-positive foetus, abortion or antepartum haemorrhage). The anti-D will coat foetal cells which are then removed from the maternal circulation before sensitization occurs. The dose of anti-D is adjusted according to the number of foetal cells detected in the maternal circulation (Kleihauer test).

Neonatal haematology

Anaemia – normal neonates have a raised Hb (16–18.5 g/dL). Premature infants are typically anaemic, and this worsens over the course of the first 6 weeks. Deficiency of iron, vitamin E and folic acid may contribute. Neonates (particularly premature) have an increased susceptibility to *infection*, though typically have normal leucocyte counts. The normal range for the *platelet count* is lower in neonates (300–400 × 10^9/L) (particularly in the premature). Important causes of neonatal thrombocytopenia are congenital infection (e.g. maternal CMV, rubella and toxoplasmosis) and neonatal alloimmune thrombocytopenia (due to transplacental passage of anti-HPA-1a, antibodies).

Haemorrhagic disease of the newborn is discussed in Chapter 39.

46 Blood transfusion I

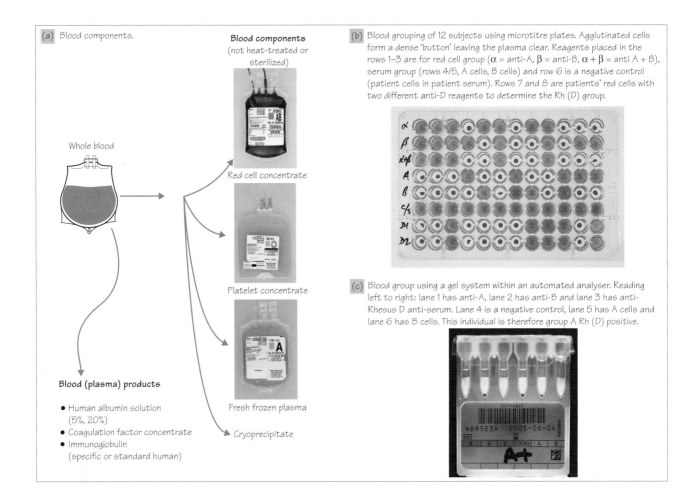

(a) Blood components.

Blood components
(not heat-treated or sterilized)

Whole blood

Red cell concentrate

Platelet concentrate

Fresh frozen plasma

Blood (plasma) products

- Human albumin solution (5%, 20%)
- Coagulation factor concentrate
- Immunoglobulin (specific or standard human)

Cryoprecipitate

(b) Blood grouping of 12 subjects using microtitre plates. Agglutinated cells form a dense 'button' leaving the plasma clear. Reagents placed in the rows 1–3 are for red cell group (α = anti-A, β = anti-B, α + β = anti A + B), serum group (rows 4/5, A cells, B cells) and row 6 is a negative control (patient cells in patient serum). Rows 7 and 8 are patients' red cells with two different anti-D reagents to determine the Rh (D) group.

(c) Blood group using a gel system within an automated analyser. Reading left to right: lane 1 has anti-A, lane 2 has anti-B and lane 3 has anti-Rhesus D anti-serum. Lane 4 is a negative control, lane 5 has A cells and lane 6 has B cells. This individual is therefore group A Rh (D) positive.

Whole blood or plasma is collected from volunteer donors. Over 90% of the donated blood is separated to allow use of individual cell components and plasma from which specific blood products can be manufactured (Fig. 46a).

In the UK, blood donors are healthy volunteers, aged 17–70 years, who are not on medication, have had no serious previous illnesses and are at low risk for transmitting infectious agents. Those who have received blood product transfusions, drug abusers, haemophiliacs, selected individuals who have recently travelled outside Europe or lived in Africa – where malaria or AIDS may be endemic – and their sexual partners are excluded. Donors are screened for anaemia and they donate two to three times each year.

Donated blood is routinely tested

- for hepatitis B and C, HIV 1 and 2, HTLV I and II, *Treponema pallidum*;
- serologically to determine the blood group (A, B or O) and Rh C, D and E type and
- selective testing for antibodies to cytomegalovirus (CMV) is used to identify donations which are CMV-negative and thus suitable for certain patients.

Blood grouping and compatibility testing
Red cells

Red cells have surface antigens which are glycoproteins or glycolipids (see Table 46.1). Individuals lacking a red cell antigen may make alloantibodies (antibodies in one individual reacting to cells of another individual) if exposed to it by transfusion or by transfer of foetal red cells across the placenta in pregnancy. Antibodies to ABO antigens occur naturally, are IgM and complete (detectable by incubation of red cells with antibody in saline at room temperature). Antibodies to other red cell antigens appear only after sensitization. They are usually IgG and incomplete, detected by special techniques, e.g. enzyme-treated red cells, addition of albumin to the reaction mixture or the indirect antiglobulin (Coombs') reaction (see Fig. 17b).

Alloantibodies may cause

- intravascular (e.g. ABO incompatibility) or extravascular (e.g. Rh incompatibility) haemolysis of donor red cells in the recipient and
- haemolytic disease of the foetus and newborn because of transplacental passage.

 Haematology at a Glance, 3e. By A. Mehta and V. Hoffbrand. Published 2009 by Blackwell Publishing. ISBN 978-1-4051-7970-6.

Table 46.1 Red cell antigens and antibodies. Incidence in UK individuals given in brackets

Cell antigens	Naturally occurring antibodies (usually IgM)	Antibodies only occurring after sensitization ('atypical' or immune (usually IgG)
A (40%)	Anti-B	
B (8%)	Anti-A	
AB (3%)	—	
O (45%)	Anti-A and Anti-B	
Rhesus (D) (85%)	—	
Rhesus cde/cde (i.e. Rh-negative) (15%)	—	Anti-D (Anti-C, Anti-c, Anti-E less common)
Kell (K) (9%)	—	anti-Kell
Duffy (Fya, Fyb) (60%)	—	anti-Duffy
Kidd (JKa, JKb) (75%)	—	anti-Kidd

NB: red cells with antigens AA or AO group as A; BB or BO group as B.

Blood grouping

An individual's red cell group is determined by suspending washed red cells with diluted anti-A, anti-B, anti-AB and anti-Rh(D). This is usually carried out in microtitre plates (Fig. 46b) or gels (Fig. 46c), but automated machines are increasingly used. Agglutination indicates a positive test. Serum is simultaneously incubated with group A, B and O cells to confirm the presence of the expected naturally occurring ABO antibodies. The recipient's serum is also incubated against a pool of group O cells which together express the most common antigens against which 'atypical' antibodies occur. If such an antibody is found, it is characterized and donor blood negative for the corresponding antigen is used for transfusion.

Compatibility testing

Compatibility testing (cross-matching) entails suspension of red cells from a donor pack with recipient serum, incubation (at room temperature and 37°C) to allow reactions to occur, and examination for agglutination, including indirect antiglobulin test (see Fig. 17b) to ensure that no reaction has occurred.

Red cell transfusion (Fig. 46a)
Indications
- Haemorrhage, severe anaemia refractory to other therapy or needing rapid correction.
- If repeated transfusions likely, phenotyped ABO and Rh(D) compatible red cells which correspond as closely as possible to the minor red cell antigens of the recipient are used to minimize sensitization.

Types of red cells
- Fresh whole blood (<5 days post-collection) is preferable for neonates.
- Red cells in optimal additive solution ('packed'), e.g. containing sodium chloride, adenine, glucose and mannitol (SAG-M) which gives red cells a shelf life of 30–35 days. These are generally used for patients with anaemia requiring red cell transfusion.
- All red cells have been passed through a leucocyte depletion filter to reduce reactions to leucocytes in patients sensitized to human leucocyte antigens (HLA) (e.g. multiply transfused patients), to reduce incidence of sensitization to HLA and to reduce risk of transmission of CMV Leucodepletion reduces the theoretical risk of transmission of new variant Creutzfeldt–Jacob disease (nvCJD, see below).

Autologous donation of red cells is suitable for some patients awaiting elective surgery. Patients donate their own red cells preoperatively on several occasions and receive iron. Donated units are screened for infectious agents in the usual way and stored at 4°C. Directed donations, e.g. within families, are not considered ethical within the UK. Salvage of autologous blood which is then washed and transfused may be carried out during major surgery, e.g. liver transplantation.

Platelet transfusion (Fig. 46a)

A single donor unit is prepared from a unit of whole blood by centrifugation within hours of collection. It contains approximately 5×10^{10} platelets in 50–60 mL fresh plasma; shelf life of 4–6 days. Standard adult dose is five pooled units and group ABO and Rh compatible, but not cross-matched, units are given. Patients with HLA may require platelets from HLA-compatible donors who have donated platelets by platelet. They are not generally used in patients with accelerated platelet destruction.

Indications
- Thrombocytopenia $<50 \times 10^9$/L – in presence of significant bleeding or prior to an invasive procedure.
- Thrombocytopenia $<10 \times 109$/L or higher in patients with infection or bleeding. Prophylactic transfustions are required in patients post-chemotherapy or stem cell transplant or with marrow failure.
- Platelet function defects (in presence of bleeding or prior to surgery), DIC (see Chapter 39) and dilutional thrombocytopenia following massive transfusion.

New drugs, e.g. which stimulate platelet production by binding with the thrombopoietin receptor cMpl on progenitor cells and megakaryocytes may well reduce requirements for platelet transfusions.

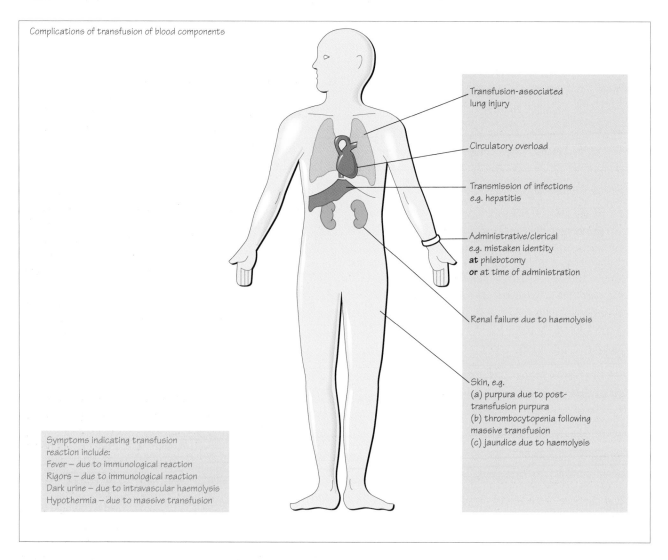

Complications of transfusion of blood components

Transfusion-associated lung injury

Circulatory overload

Transmission of infections e.g. hepatitis

Administrative/clerical e.g. mistaken identity **at** phlebotomy **or** at time of administration

Renal failure due to haemolysis

Skin, e.g.
(a) purpura due to post-transfusion purpura
(b) thrombocytopenia following massive transfusion
(c) jaundice due to haemolysis

Symptoms indicating transfusion reaction include:
Fever – due to immunological reaction
Rigors – due to immunological reaction
Dark urine – due to intravascular haemolysis
Hypothermia – due to massive transfusion

Fresh frozen plasma

Fresh frozen plasma (FFP) is a source of all coagulation and other plasma proteins. Compatibility testing is not required, but blood group compatible units are used. FFP from group AB donors may be used if the recipient blood group is unknown. As FFP is not heat sterilized and may transmit infection, solvent-treated FFP may be safer in this regard.

Indications

• Coagulation factor replacement. Perform coagulation tests and platelet count prior to use. Patients with disseminated intravascular coagulation (DIC) or massive transfusion at risk of bleeding and with coagulation abnormalities may benefit. Single-factor deficiencies are best treated with a specific factor concentrate.
• Liver disease – in the presence of bleeding or prior to invasive procedures, e.g. liver biopsy; combined with vitamin K.

• Haemolytic uraemic syndrome or thrombotic thrombocytopenic purpura usually with plasma exchange. Cryoprecipitate-poor FFP is preferred.
• Reversal of oral anticoagulation or thrombolytic therapy.

Cryoprecipitate

Cryoprecipitate is prepared from the precipitate formed from FFP during controlled thawing, resuspended in 20-mL plasma. It is rich in fibrinogen, fibronectin and factor VIII. Group compatible units are used. It may be useful in patients with DIC, liver disease, following massive transfusion and, rarely, in von Willebrand's disease.

Other blood products

These are derived from pooled human plasma which has undergone a manufacturing process designed to concentrate and sterilize the component. They carry a theoretical risk of transmitting diseases caused by prions (e.g. nvCJD). There have been no fully documented cases of this with blood products other than red cell transfusions, but the current UK practice is to use products made by recombinant DNA or plasma from non-UK donors.

Coagulation factor concentrates

Coagulation factor concentrates are available as freeze-dried powder of high purity. Factor VIII concentrate is used for treatment of haemophilia A and von Willebrand's disease; recombinant factor VIII is now available. Factor IX concentrate, also available as recombinant, is used in patients with haemophilia B. Factor IX complex (prothrombin complex) also contains factors II, VII and X and is of value in patients with specific disorders involving factors II and X, oral anticoagulant overdose, in severe liver failure and to overcome inhibitors to factor VIII in patients with haemophilia A who have developed inhibitors. Its use carries a risk of provoking thrombosis and DIC.

Other concentrates include protein C, antithrombin, factors VII, XI and XIII and are used in the corresponding congenital deficiencies. Protein C concentrate is also used in severe DIC, e.g. meningococcal septicaemia.

Recombinant human factor VIIa

This may be used for patients with massive uncontrollable haemorrhage post-trauma and surgery. It may cause thrombosis. It is extremely expensive.

Albumin solution

Albumin solution is available as 5, 20 and 20 salt-poor formulations. It contains no coagulation factors. It is used in the treatment of hypovolaemia, particularly when caused by burns, and shock associated with multiple organ failure. Synthetic plasma volume expanders (e.g. dextrans, gelatin and hydroxyethyl starch) are of equal value in initial management. These 'colloids' remain longer within the intravascular space than 'crystalloid' solutions (e.g. 0.9% NaCl), exert a colloid osmotic effect and may elevate blood pressure. Resistant oedema in patients with renal and hepatic disease requires 20% albumin.

Immunoglobulins

Immunoglobulins (Igs) are prepared from pooled donor plasma by fractionation and sterile filtration. Specific Igs include hepatitis B and herpes zoster, which provide passive immune protection. Standard human Ig for intramuscular injection is used for prophylaxis against hepatitis A, rubella and measles, whereas hyperimmune globulin is prepared from donors with high titres of the relevant antibodies for prophylaxis of tetanus, hepatitis A, diphtheria, rabies, mumps, measles, rubella, cytomegalovirus and *Pseudomonas* infections. Intravenous Ig may be used to protect against infections in patients with congenital or acquired immune deficiency and in high doses is of value in some autoimmune disorders, e.g. immune thrombocytopenic purpura, Guillain–Barre syndrome.

White cell transfusion

White cell (buffy coat) transfusions are now rarely used in neutropenic patients as there are few data demonstrating clinical efficacy.

Complications of transfusion (see Fig. 47)

- **Administrative and clerical errors** must be avoided by rigorous adherence to procedures for checking and documentation when ordering, prescribing, issuing and administering blood components. **These are by far the most common cause of serious and 'near miss' incidents**.
- **Congestive heart failure** caused by circulatory overload.
- **Immunological reactions** may occur with transfusion of cellular and plasma-derived blood components. ABO-incompatible red cell transfusions may lead to life-threatening intravascular haemolysis of transfused cells with fever, rigors, haemoglobinuria, hypotension and renal failure. Atypical antibodies arising from previous transfusions or pregnancy may cause intravascular or, more commonly, delayed extravascular haemolysis with anaemia, jaundice, splenomegaly and fever.

Hypersensitivity reactions to plasma components may cause urticaria, wheezing, facial oedema and pyrexia but can cause anaphylactic shock, especially in IgA-deficient subjects.

Treatment

The transfusion must be stopped immediately. For severe reactions, the clerical details must be checked and samples from the donor unit and recipient are analysed for compatibility and haemolysis. Recipient serum is analysed for presence of atypical red cell, leucocyte, HLA and plasma protein antibodies. Support care to maintain blood pressure and renal function and to promote diuresis and treat shock (intravenous steroids, antihistamines, adrenaline in severe cases) may be necessary.

- **Transmission of infection.** *Bacterial infections* can occur through failure of sterile technique at the time of collection or because of bacteraemia in the donor. *Protozoal infections* (e.g. malaria) can be transmitted and at-risk donors are not eligible to donate. *Viral infection* can be transmitted in spite of mandatory screening, as seroconversion may not have occurred in an infected donor, the virus may not have been identified, or the most sensitive serological tests may not be routinely performed (e.g. testing for antihepatitis B core antibodies). The risk of transmission is much lower for those blood products which have undergone a manufacturing and sterilization process. There are a few documented cases of transmission of nvCJD by red cell transfusions.
- **Other complications.** Iron overload occurs in multiply transfused patients (see Chapter 12). Graft versus host disease may be caused by transfusion of viable T lymphocytes into severely immunosuppressed hosts, so cellular components should be irradiated prior to transfusion to foetuses, premature neonates, stem cell transplantation recipients, patients who have received fludarabine and other severely immunocompromised patients.

48 Stem cell transplantation

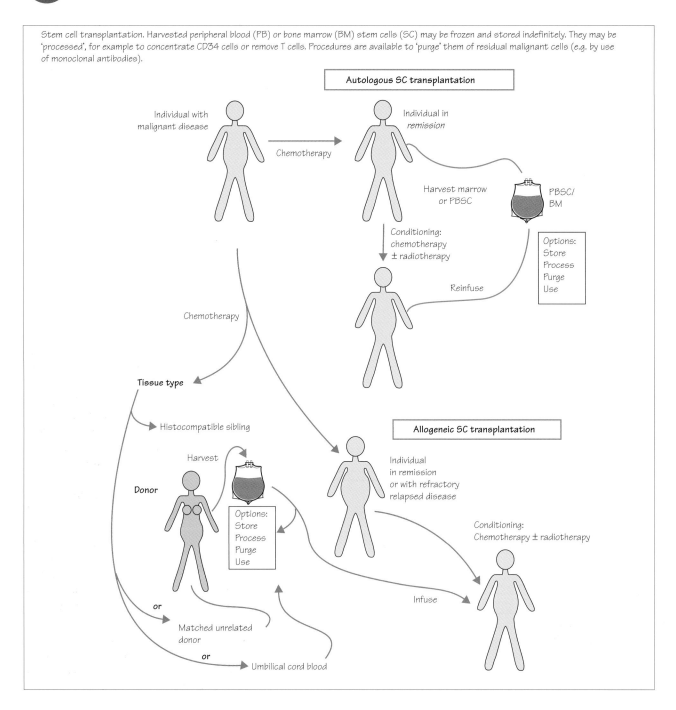

Stem cell transplantation. Harvested peripheral blood (PB) or bone marrow (BM) stem cells (SC) may be frozen and stored indefinitely. They may be 'processed', for example to concentrate CD34 cells or remove T cells. Procedures are available to 'purge' them of residual malignant cells (e.g. by use of monoclonal antibodies).

Autologous SC transplantation

Individual with malignant disease
Chemotherapy
Individual in remission
Harvest marrow or PBSC
PBSC/ BM
Conditioning: chemotherapy ± radiotherapy
Reinfuse
Options: Store Process Purge Use

Chemotherapy
Tissue type
Histocompatible sibling
Harvest
Donor
Options: Store Process Purge Use
or
Matched unrelated donor
or
Umbilical cord blood

Allogeneic SC transplantation

Individual in remission or with refractory relapsed disease
Conditioning: Chemotherapy ± radiotherapy
Infuse

Stem cell transplantation (SCT) (see figure above) is the use of haemopoietic stem cells (HSC) from a donor harvested from peripheral blood (peripheral blood stem cells, PBSC) or bone marrow, to repopulate recipient bone marrow.

• **Allogeneic** SCT involves transplantation of HSC from one individual to another. This is usually between two HLA matching individuals, most frequently siblings but, in their absence, volunteer and HLA-matched unrelated donors (MUD) are increasingly being used. HLA matching includes class I (A, B) and class II (DR) tested by molecular typing. If the donor is

an identical twin, the transplant is termed 'syngeneic'. Conventional allogeneic SCT is rarely performed in individuals >60 years of age, as it carries risk of treatment-related morbidity and even mortality (up to 5–10%) which increases with age. 'Mini-' or low-intensity transplants in which the recipient receives immunosuppressive but not myeloablative therapy are preferred for older recipients (>60 yr) as the pre-transplant conditioning is less intensive and the procedure is safer in older patients.

• **Autologous** SCT utilizes the patient's own stem cells. These are harvested from the patient and then used to repopulate the

Table 48.1 Conditions for which stem cell transplantation has been used

Allogeneic	Autologous
Acute leukaemia and ALL	**Selected patients with**
Chronic or accelerated phase CML	Myeloma
Severe aplastic anaemia	Lymphoma
	Autoimmune disease,
	e.g. scleroderma
Myelodysplasia	
Lymphoma	
Myeloma	
Chronic lymphocytic leukaemia	
Thalassaemia major, sickle cell	
disease	
Severe inherited metabolic	
diseases, e.g. adenosine	
deaminase deficiency and	
Hurler's syndrome	

ALL, acute lymphoblastic leukaemia; AML, acute myeloid leukaemia; CML, chronic myeloid leukaemia

marrow after further high-dose chemotherapy and/or radiotherapy. Autologous SCT may be performed more safely in older patients, up to 70 years.
• **Cord** blood transplantation utilizes foetal stem cells harvested at the time of birth from the umbilical cord.

Indications

SCT is used in the hope of curing or substantially prolonging remission in patients with a wide variety of haematological and other diseases. For allogeneic or autologous SCT, the recipient requires 'conditioning' therapy (chemotherapy ± radiotherapy) pre-transplant to help eradicate malignant disease in bone marrow and elsewhere and to cause immunosuppression, thereby reducing risk of marrow rejection in the case of allogeneic SCT. Stem cells (donor or recipients own) are then infused to rescue the patient from bone marrow failure. The transplanted immune system in an allogeneic SCT may itself have antitumour, e.g. graft versus leukaemia (GVL) effect, and this is the major way in which allogeneic SCT whether 'mini' or with full conditioning eliminates the malignant disease (Table 48.1).

Procedure

Treatment with a haemopoietic growth factor (e.g. G-CSF), combined in the case of autologous SCT with chemotherapy,

e.g. high-dose cyclophosphamide, is used to mobilize HSC from bone marrow into peripheral blood, where they are collected by leucopheresis. Alternatively, HSC may be harvested from marrow by multiple bone marrow aspirations, performed under general anaesthesia. Approximately 2×10^8/kg nucleated cells or 2×10^6/kg CD34 cells are needed (CD34 is a surface marker of early haemopoietic stem and progenitor cells). The recipient of an allogeneic or MUD transplant then receives immunosuppressive drugs to reduce the risk of graft versus host disease (GVHD) (see below).

Complications

Complications of SCT include the following:
• Side effects of conditioning chemotherapy/radiotherapy, e.g. bone marrow failure, nausea, alopecia, skin burns, pulmonary toxicity, hepatic veno-occlusive disease, toxicity to endocrine organs and growth retardation.
• Rejection of transplanted HSC.
• Relapse of original disease. This is sometimes treated by infusion of lymphocytes from the allogeneic donor, which will have a GVL effect.
• Infection following SCT occurs because patients are severely immunosuppressed. Infection may be bacterial, viral, protozoal or fungal. Prophylactic antibiotic, antifungal and antiviral therapy is given. Cytomegalovirus (CMV)-negative recipients should receive blood components which are leucodepleted or from CMV-negative donors. CMV infection may cause pneumonitis, diarrhoea, liver dysfunction, skin rash and graft failure, and is a major cause of transplant-related mortality. Ganciclovir and foscarnet are useful in treatment of CMV infection. Prophylaxis against *Pneumocystis carinii* infection is with oral co-trimoxazole and/or nebulized pentamidine.
• Metabolic problems, often caused by multiple intravenous drugs (antibiotics, antivirals, antifungals), renal failure, blood component therapy, intravenous feeding, etc.
• GVHD (allogeneic SCT). Transplanted lymphocytes may recognize the recipient as 'foreign' and mount an immunological onslaught, to cause skin rash, liver disease and diarrhoea. The incidence of GVHD is higher in older patients. Acute GVHD (<100 days after SCT) typically begins 7–10 days after transplantation and is graded according to severity. Chronic GVHD (>100 days) presents with a scleroderma-like syndrome with liver, lung, gastrointestinal or joint abnormalities. The incidence and severity of GVHD may be decreased by depleting T cells from donor marrow and immune suppression of the recipient, e.g. with cyclosporin and methotrexate.

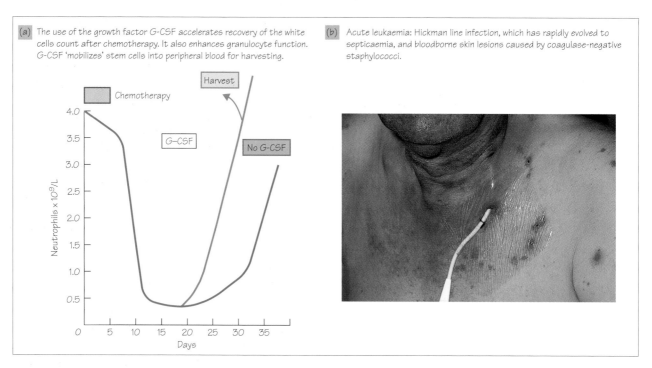

(a) The use of the growth factor G-CSF accelerates recovery of the white cells count after chemotherapy. It also enhances granulocyte function. G-CSF 'mobilizes' stem cells into peripheral blood for harvesting.

(b) Acute leukaemia: Hickman line infection, which has rapidly evolved to septicaemia, and bloodborne skin lesions caused by coagulase-negative staphylococci.

Chemotherapy

Chemotherapy is the use of pharmacological agents (Table 49.1) to treat malignant or other proliferative diseases. It may be given orally, by intravenous bolus, prolonged subcutaneous or intravenous injection/infusion or intrathecally. It may be a single agent or combination of chemotherapy-utilizing drugs with different, preferably synergistic, modes of action, with limited or no overlapping toxicity, and aimed at delaying emergence of drug resistance. Chemotherapy drugs are often given as a cycle of a few days' treatment every 3–6 weeks to allow normal cells, especially of the bone marrow and gastrointestinal tract, to recover from toxicity. Extravasation into tissues can cause severe local reactions. Intravenous chemotherapy is usually given through a central line or through a tunnelled intravenous catheter (e.g. Hickman's) or indwelling chamber (e.g. Porta-Cath).

Mechanism of action

Chemotherapy drugs generally affect DNA synthesis or repair and promote cellular apoptosis. Cycle-specific agents prevent DNA synthesis and act on the S phase of the cell cycle (Table 49.1). Non-cycle-specific agents act at all phases of the cell cycle and include alkylating agents, which bind to DNA, and anthracyclines, which cause DNA strand breaks. Inhibition of the DNA repair enzyme, topoisomerase II, is an important component of the action of anthracyclines and etoposide.

Side-effects of chemotherapy - see Chapter 50.

Biological therapies

Growth factors in clinical use (see Chapter 1) include granulocyte colony-stimulating factor (Fig. 49a), erythropoietin and synthetic analogues of thrombopoietin. The interferons are nat-

urally occurring agents which have both antineoplastic and anti-infective properties. Monoclonal antibodies, e.g. rituximab (anti-CD20), alemtuzumab (anti-CD52) and Mylotarg (anti-CD33), alone or bound to toxins or radioactive isotopes may be used to kill specific cells or target drug therapy. Thalidomide and lenalidomide are used to treat myeloma, myelodysplasia and myelofibrosis.

Infection

The main risk factors are
• neutropenia (particularly if $<0.5 \times 10^9$/L) for bacterial and fungal infections;
• organisms which are normal commensals may be pathogenic for immunocompromised patients;
• defective cell-mediated or humoral immunity for viral, bacterial and atypical infections (e.g. tuberculosis);
• others, such as indwelling catheters (intravenous, urethral), corticosteroid therapy and mucositis, also increase risk. Impaired splenic function or splenectomy reduce ability to make antibody, particularly to capsulated organisms, reduces clearance of intracellular organisms (e.g. parasitized red cells) and impairs defence against organisms and toxins in the portal circulation.

Organisms

These include the following:
• bacterial – gram-positive (coagulase-negative and -positive staphylococci, streptococci, enterococci); gram-negative (*Klebsiella*, *Pseudomonas*, *Escherichia coli*, *Proteus*); others, e.g. tuberculosis, atypical mycobacteria (Fig. 49b);
• fungal – *Candida*, *Aspergillus*;

Table 49.1 Chemotherapy agents

DNA binding

Anthracyclines	Other
Daunorubicin	Mitoxantrone
Hydroxydaunorubicin	Bleomycin
Idarubicin	

Alkylating agents

Cyclophosphamide	Melphalan
Ifosphamide	Nitrosoureas (BCNU, CCNU)
Chlorambucil	Busulphan

Mitotic inhibitors
Vincristine
Vindesine
Vinblastine

Antimetabolites

Methotrexate	Cytosine arabinoside
Mercaptopurine	Hydroxyurea
Thioguanine	

Inhibitors of DNA repair enzymes
Epipodophyllotoxins

Antipurines
Fludarabine
Deoxycoformycin
2-Chlorodeoxydenosine

Others
Corticosteroids
L-Asparaginase
Biological agents: Interferon, Thalidomide

Monoclonal antibodies

Rituximab	anti-CD20
Alemtuzimab	anti-CD52
Mylotarg	anti-CD33
Zevalin	anti-CD20
Ecluzimab	anti-complement C5

- viruses – cytomegalovirus, herpes viruses, adenoviruses and
- protozoans – *Toxoplasma, Pneumocystis, Leishmania, Histoplasma.*

Prevention

- Good hygiene on the part of the patient and staff, regular hand cleaning and avoidance of contact with infected individuals.
- Barrier nursing in isolation is preferred. Staff wear gowns and gloves when in contact with severely neutropenic patients.
- Filtered air at positive pressure reduces risk from fungal spores.
- Food should ideally be cooked. Foods frequently contaminated with bacteria (soft cheeses, uncooked eggs and meat, salads, live yoghurt) are avoided and only peeled fruits are allowed.
- Oral non-absorbable antibiotics (e.g. neomycin, colistin) will reduce colonization of the gastrointestinal tract; oral systemic antibiotics (ciprofloxacin, co-trimoxazole) reduce the incidence of bacteraemia and oral antifungals (fluconazole/amphotericin/itraconazole/posaconazole) and/or oral antiviral

(aciclovir) prophylaxis are routinely given in some units for selected patients.

Diagnosis

- Fever is the cardinal sign of infection; tachycardia, tachypnoea, fall in blood pressure, cough, dysuria and altered mental state may also occur.
- Physical signs include reddened throat, inflamed intravenous catheter site, skin rash, chest signs, mouth signs and perineal inflammation. Pus is absent in neutropenic patients.
- Special tests to identify the responsible organism include microbial culture (sputum, urine, throat and perineal swab, blood cultures from peripheral blood and indwelling catheter, lumbar puncture – if neurological symptoms – skin swabs, faecal culture). Bronchoalveolar lavage may be necessary. Serological and molecular tests for specific organisms, e.g. *Candida, Aspergillus,* may be of value. Imaging tests may include chest X-ray, CT scan, especially of chest if fungal infection is suspected, and sinus X-rays.

Treatment

- Supportive care for renal failure/hypotension/respiratory failure.
- Empirical antibacterial therapy should be commenced in patients who are neutropenic ($<0.5 \times 10^9$/L) or otherwise severely immunocompromised and develop fever (temperature of 38 °C or greater lasting for more than 2 h). Cultures should be taken and intravenous antibiotics should be commenced, with either a single, potent broad-spectrum agent (e.g. a fourth-generation cephalosporin or ureidopenicillin) or a combination of agents with activity against gram-negative and gram-positive (including coagulase negative staphylococci) organisms.
- Failure to respond should prompt treatment of atypical infections, e.g. fungi, viruses. Empirical antifungal treatment with liposomal amphotericin/voriconozole/caspofungin is required in high-risk patients, particularly after stem cell transplantation.

Radiotherapy

Ionizing radiation, usually derived from an external source, is used to treat disease by causing DNA damage in malignant cells. It is commonly used in the treatment of haematological malignancies (e.g. lymphoid leukaemias, lymphoma, myeloma) and as part of conditioning therapy for bone marrow transplant for malignant disease. Side effects include nausea, vomiting, alopecia, bone marrow failure, damage to normal tissues (e.g. skin burns), growth retardation and induction of second malignancies.

Counselling

Counselling is valuable for various groups of haematological patients.

- Patients and families with malignant disease need emotional support during treatment and/or bereavement. Practical help with housing, transport, welfare benefits, etc should also be given. There should be good liaison with GPs, palliative and terminal care support teams in the community and hospices.
- Genetic counselling is needed in families with haemophilia, genetic disorders of haemoglobin and thrombophilia.

50 Haematological effects of drugs

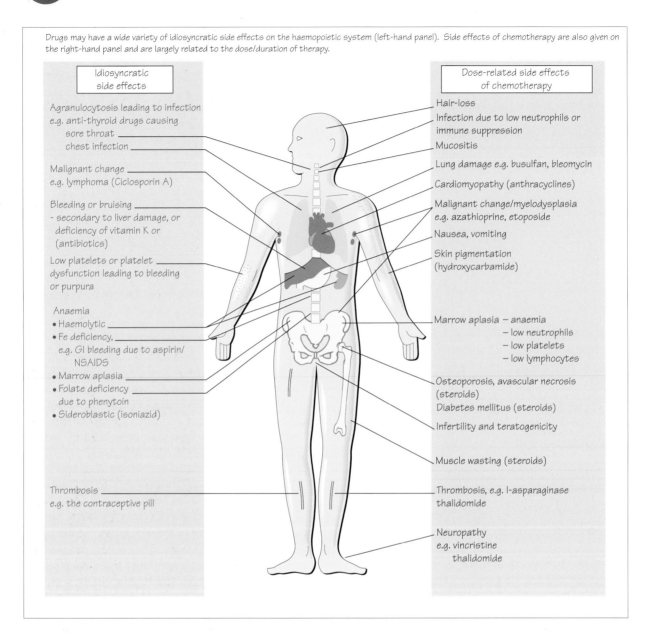

Drugs may have a wide variety of idiosyncratic side effects on the haemopoietic system (left-hand panel). Side effects of chemotherapy are also given on the right-hand panel and are largely related to the dose/duration of therapy.

Idiosyncratic side effects

Agranulocytosis leading to infection e.g. anti-thyroid drugs causing sore throat chest infection

Malignant change e.g. lymphoma (Ciclosporin A)

Bleeding or bruising - secondary to liver damage, or deficiency of vitamin K or (antibiotics)

Low platelets or platelet dysfunction leading to bleeding or purpura

Anaemia
• Haemolytic
• Fe deficiency, e.g. GI bleeding due to aspirin/NSAIDS
• Marrow aplasia
• Folate deficiency due to phenytoin
• Sideroblastic (isoniazid)

Thrombosis e.g. the contraceptive pill

Dose-related side effects of chemotherapy

Hair-loss

Infection due to low neutrophils or immune suppression

Mucositis

Lung damage e.g. busulfan, bleomycin

Cardiomyopathy (anthracyclines)

Malignant change/myelodysplasia e.g. azathioprine, etoposide

Nausea, vomiting

Skin pigmentation (hydroxycarbamide)

Marrow aplasia – anaemia
– low neutrophils
– low platelets
– low lymphocytes

Osteoporosis, avascular necrosis (steroids)

Diabetes mellitus (steroids)

Infertility and teratogenicity

Muscle wasting (steroids)

Thrombosis, e.g. l-asparaginase thalidomide

Neuropathy e.g. vincristine thalidomide

Drugs may cause a wide variety of haematological changes. Two broad categories of effect occur:
• Idiosyncratic – i.e. effects which occur only in certain individuals and are independent of the dose.
• Dose-dependent and predictable effects.

Genetic mechanisms may underlie individual susceptibility to side effects. Genetic traits may also influence drug metabolism – e.g. some individuals metabolise purines such that certain drugs (azathioprine) are more likely to cause bone marrow suppression.

Recognising, monitoring and reporting haematologic toxicity is an important parts are of the marketing and post-marketing surveillance and assessment of new drugs. Mechanisms of haematologic toxicity include:

• Direct toxicity of the drug or its metabolites to haemopoietic stem cells or more mature cells;
• Induction of immune-mediated damage to haematologic stem cells;
• Effects on intermediary metabolism of haematinics or vitamins;
• Indirect effects via damage to other organs, e.g. the liver;
• Predisposition to malignant change.

Side effects of chemotherapy
Most chemotherapeutic agents are toxic to normal dividing cells (haemopoietic cells, gastrointestinal tract, hair, skin) as well as to malignant cells. Common side effects include the following:

- Bone marrow failure (anaemia, thrombocytopenia, leucopenia) with increased susceptibility to bleeding and infection, which may require therapy with antimicrobials, blood components and growth factors (G-CSF, erythropoietin) and synthetic thrombomimetics.
- Nausea and vomiting, requiring antiemetic therapy – metoclopramide, dexamethasone and 5-HT antagonists (e.g. ondansetron, granisetron).
- Mucositis (sore mouth and throat), abdominal pain and diarrhoea.
- Infertility – sperm storage considered *before* chemotherapy.
- Tumour lysis syndrome – prevented by good hydration, alkalinization of urine, allopurinol.
- Hyperuricaemia – prevented by allopurinol.
- Specific side effects of chemotherapy include neuropathy (vincristine), cardiomyopathy (anthracyclines), thrombosis (L-asparaginase), pulmonary fibrosis (busulphan, bleomycin) and haemorrhagic cystitis (cyclophosphamide).
- Secondary malignancy, e.g. myelodysplasia or acute leukaemia following alkylating agents or etoposide.
- Growth retardation in children.

Stem cell damage

- Pancytopenia occurs in a *predictable* dose-dependent fashion following chemotherapy or radiotherapy involving the bone marrow. Chemotherapeutic agents which particularly induce marrow hypocellularity include anthracyclines, epipodophyllotoxins, alkylating agents and antimetabolitis.
- *Idiosyncratic* aplastic anaemia occurs rarely (e.g. 1 in 20,000–100,000 individuals exposed to the same drug) and is independent of the dose. Drugs with this potential side effect include antibiotics (e.g. chloramphenicol, sulphonamides), anti-rheumatic drugs (e.g. gold, indomethacin) and chlorpromazine. It is typically severe, up to 50% of patients do not recover their blood counts, and may require treatment for bone marrow failure (see Chapter 20).

Anaemia

The commonest form of drug-induced anaemia is iron deficiency due to blood loss. Aspirin, non-steroidal anti-inflammatory drugs (NSAIDS) and corticosteroids can all cause bleeding from the upper gastrointestinal tract. Iron absorption is impaired by tetracyclines. Megaloblastic anaemia due to folate deficiency may complicate treatment with anti-epilepsy (e.g. phenytoin) and other drugs. Some drugs, e.g. isoniazid, antagonise vitamin B_6 and sideroblastic anaemia by acting as competitive antagonists.

Drug-induced haemolytic anaemias

These may be immune or non-immune.

Immune mechanisms include the following:
- Antibody directed against the drug, e.g. penicillin–red cell membrane complex, the drug acting as a hapten.
- Antibody against a drug, e.g. quinidine–plasma protein complex with subsequent deposition of the immune complex on red cells.
- Stimulation of autoantibody (warm type) production against the red cell, e.g. methyldopa.

Non-immune mechanisms include the following:
- Haemolysis in G6PD-deficient individuals (many drugs, see Chapter 16).
- Haemolysis in normal individuals, e.g. dapsone.

White cells

Agranulocytosis may occur as part of aplastic anaemia or in isolation. Idiosyncratic agranulocytosis is seen with anti-thyroid drugs, e.g. carbimazole, deferiprone (up to 1% of all recipients), anti-psychotic drugs, e.g. Clozaril and antibiotics (sulphonamide, tetracycline). Eosinophilia may be seen as part of an allergic reaction to virtually any drug.

Platelets

Drugs can cause an increased risk of bruising and bleeding by interfering with platelet function, e.g. aspirin and NSAIDS, which inhibit prostaglandin synthesis. Thrombocytopenia may occur as an immune phenomenon, e.g. due to sulphonamides, thiazide diuretics, quinine or due to direct toxicity, alone or as part of aplastic anaemia, e.g. thiazides, sulphonamides.

Coagulation factors

Alterations may lead to increased risk of bleeding, e.g. aspirin-induced hypofibrinogenaemia; or prolonged antibiotic therapy, causing impaired vitamin K absorption. Alternatively, an increased risk of thrombosis occurs during prolonged antibiotic therapy. The contraceptive pill (oestrogens) may cause an increase in coagulation factors and a reduction in circulating levels of coagulation inhibitors, e.g. protein S.

Drug-induced malignant change

Myelodysplasia may occur following prolonged use of alkylating agents combination chemotherapy for acute leukaemia or lymphoma. MPS or non-Hodgkin lymphoma may occur following immunosuppressive therapy, e.g. cyclosporine A or azathioprine, which can cause Epstein–Barr virus-associated lymphoproliferative disorders, particularly after transplantation; lymphoma has also been reported following phenytoin therapy.

MCQs

1 Iron deficiency anaemia
   (a) Is usually associated with a raised MCV.
   (b) The MCH is usually low.
   (c) Is most commonly due to dietary deficiency.
   (d) Is associated with a low serum ferritin.
   (e) Responds much more quickly to parenteral than oral therapy.

2 Macrocytic anaemia
   (a) Occurs in renal failure.
   (b) May result from vitamin B_{12} deficiency.
   (c) Occurs in the context of chronic inflammatory disease.
   (d) May be associated with myxoedema.
   (e) May be associated with thalassemia.

3 Chronic myeloid leukaemia
   (a) Is the commonest form of leukaemia worldwide.
   (b) Usually presents with bone marrow failure.
   (c) Is usually associated with the presence of the Philadelphia chromosome.
   (d) May respond to treatment with interferon.
   (e) Usually transforms to an acute leukaemia.

4 Chronic lymphocytic leukaemia
   (a) Is a cause of hypogammaglobulinaemia.
   (b) Is commonly treated with intensive combination chemotherapy.
   (c) Is associated with a median survival of <2 years.
   (d) Often presents asymptomatically.
   (e) Is more commonly derived from B cells than T cells.

5 The myelodysplastic syndrome (MDS)
   (a) May occur as a result of prior chemotherapy.
   (b) Is thought to have a viral aetiology.
   (c) May be associated with the presence of ring sideroblasts.
   (d) May be associated with pancytopenia.
   (e) Is characterized by a reduction in the circulating monocyte count.

6 With regard to anticoagulant therapy
   (a) Warfarin is safer than heparin in pregnancy.
   (b) The INR is used to control heparin therapy.
   (c) Low-molecular-weight heparin can be given orally.
   (d) Vitamin K is used to reverse the action of warfarin.
   (e) Should be undertaken lifelong after a single pulmonary embolus.

7 Fresh frozen plasma
   (a) Is recommended in the treatment of haemophilia A.
   (b) Is heat treated and therefore free from risk of transmission of viral disease.
   (c) Is useful in the treatment of immune thrombocytopenia.
   (d) Is useful in the treatment of thrombotic thrombocytopenic purpura.
   (e) Must be prepared from whole blood within a few hours of donation.

8 Neonatal thrombocytopenia
   (a) Can occur in infants of mothers with immune thrombocytopenia.
   (b) Is often due to intrauterine viral infection.
   (c) May be due to transplacental passage of anti-platelet antibodies from the mother.
   (d) Often improves spontaneously.
   (e) May be associated with absent radii.

9 Haemolytic anaemia
   (a) Occurs whenever red cell survival is reduced.
   (b) Is often accompanied by an increase in serum unconjugated bilirubin.
   (c) Is usually accompanied by increased urinary bilirubin.
   (d) Is predominantly extravascular in hereditary spherocytosis.
   (e) Can lead to kernicterus in the neonate.

10 An increase in peripheral blood eosinophils (eosinophilia)
   (a) Is commonly seen in bacterial infection.
   (b) May be an indicator of drug hypersensitivity.
   (c) Is commonly seen in myeloproliferative disorders.
   (d) Can lead to cardiomyopathy.
   (e) Can occur in connective tissue disorders.

11 Haematological changes during normal pregnancy include
   (a) An increase in mean corpuscular volume.
   (b) An increased incidence of thalassaemia trait.
   (c) Increased circulating levels of factor VIII.
   (d) Neutrophilia.
   (e) Increased platelet count.

12 Polycythaemia rubra vera
   (a) Occurs more frequently in smokers.
   (b) May present as gout.
   (c) Many transform to acute leukaemia.
   (d) Is frequently associated with raised white cell and platelet counts.
   (e) Is associated with an enlarged spleen.

13 Platelets
   (a) Are important sources of thrombin.
   (b) Are often multinucleated.
   (c) Are often increased in number in patients with iron deficiency.
   (d) Will aggregate in response to ADP.
   (e) Are sometimes reduced in number in von Willebrand's disease.

14 Haemopoietic stem cells
   (a) Are derived from the thymus.
   (b) Circulate in peripheral blood.
   (c) Are progenitors for plasma cells.
   (d) Do not express the CD34 antigen.
   (e) Decline in number with increasing age.

15 With regard to autosomal recessive conditions
   (a) Glucose-6-phosphate dehydrogenase deficiency is an example.
   (b) Hereditary spherocytosis is an example.

(c) There is a 1:2 chance that the offspring of two carriers will be homozygous.

(d) The carrier state may be associated with a small survival advantage.

(e) There is usually a disease-related mutation within a single gene.

16 The following are known to cause aplastic anaemia

(a) Chloramphenicol therapy.

(b) Malaria.

(c) Amyloidosis.

(d) Viral hepatitis.

(e) Renal cysts.

17 With regard to stem cell transplantation (SCT)

(a) Allogeneic SCT is indicated for all patients with AML in first remission who have an HLA-identical sibling.

(b) Matched unrelated donor (MUD) transplantation is contraindicated in children.

(c) The incidence of graft versus host disease (GVHD) is reduced by depletion of T cells from the graft.

(d) Donor stem cells are irradiated to reduce GVHD.

(e) EBV infection is a major cause of post-transplant mortality.

18 The non-Hodgkin lymphomas

(a) Are more likely to be T-cell than B-cell lineage.

(b) Occur more frequently in patients with HIV infection.

(c) Are more likely to be disseminated (stage IV) when the histology is of indolent disease than when histology shows aggressive disease.

(d) Are more common than Hodgkin lymphoma.

(e) Are declining in incidence.

19 The following are risk factors for thrombosis

(a) Haemophilia B.

(b) Resistance is activated protein C.

(c) Nephrotic syndrome.

(d) Raised levels of plasma homocysteine.

(e) Paroxysmal nocturnal haemoglobinuria.

20 Important causes of humoral immunodeficiency include

(a) Pyruvate kinase deficiency.

(b) Multiple myeloma.

(c) Indolent non-Hodgkin lymphoma.

(d) Lymphadenopathy.

(e) Presence of factor V Leiden.

21 Disseminated intravascular coagulation

(a) Is commonly seen as a presenting feature of acute promyelocytic leukaemia.

(b) Is usually associated with a raised platelet count.

(c) Is usually associated with reduced fibrinogen levels.

(d) Is usually associated with a prolonged APTT.

(e) Is usually associated with a normal thrombin time.

22 Features suggesting a population of haemopoietic cells are monoclonal include

(a) Reactive proliferation in response to infection.

(b) Uniform presence of an oncogene mutation.

(c) Demonstration of a common chromosomal abnormality.

(d) Positive staining for CD13 antigen.

(e) Presence of Howell–Jolly bodies.

23 Thrombin

(a) Is activated by heparin.

(b) Promotes platelet aggregation.

(c) Causes deficient platelet aggregation in von Willebrand's disease.

(d) Is cross-linked by Factor XIII.

(e) Is cleaved by plasmin.

24 Protein C

(a) Levels are reduced in vitamin K deficiency.

(b) Deficiency predisposes to skin necrosis after commencing oral anticoagulant therapy.

(c) Levels are inversely related to protein S levels.

(d) Levels are reduced in liver disease.

(e) Deficiency is a risk factor for thrombosis.

25 Acute leukaemia in children

(a) Is more likely to be lymphoid than myeloid.

(b) Has a remission rate following chemotherapy of <50%.

(c) Is more common in children with Down syndrome.

(d) Carries a worse prognosis if presenting WBC is $>50 \times 10^9/L$.

(e) May present with lytic bone lesions.

Case studies and questions

Case 1

A 66-year-old Caucasian man gives a history of increasing tiredness and lethargy over the preceding 2–4 months. He has recently lost his wife and has been drinking more alcohol than usual. His appetite is poor and he has lost 1 stone weight over the past 3 months. He eats a mixed diet. His bowels are regular and he does not report any blood loss. He is not on any medication. He has not had any illnesses in the past.

On examination, he is pale but not jaundiced. His blood pressure is 135/80. Abdominal examination, including rectal, is normal and there are no other abnormalities.

His FBC shows:

Hb = 7.6 g/dL
MCV = 68 fl
MCH = 26
WBC = 8.6×10^9/L
Platelets = 490×10^9/L
ESR = 83 mm/h

1 *What is the differential diagnosis?*
2 *How would you manage him?*

Case 2

A 71-year-old man has back pain. This has been present for over 3 months and is worse in the lower back. He has also developed upper abdominal pain and constipation over the last month. He has had no serious illnesses in the past. His appetite is poor and he has lost 1 stone weight over the previous month. His medication includes painkillers (paracetamol and Ibuprofen).

On examination, he is pale. His blood pressure is slightly elevated (160/100). Urine examination shows 2+ proteinuria.

Investigations show:

Hb = 8.6 g/dL
WBC = 9.5×10^9/L
Platelets = 65×10^9/L
ESR = 110 mm/h
Blood film report: Rouleaux
Leucoerythroblastic changes present

1 *What is the differential diagnosis?*
2 *What further tests are indicated?*

Case 3

A 64-year-old Caucasian woman complains of gradually increasing tiredness. She feels the cold more than she used to. She also has a sore tongue. Over the past 2 months, she has complained of numbness of her feet. Her sister suffers from hypothyroidism. She eats a normal diet.

On examination, she is pale and slightly jaundiced. Her tongue is reddened and enlarged; she has grey hair. The thyroid gland is clinically normal. She has reduced touch and joint position sense in the toes and the ankle jerks are absent. Neurological examination is otherwise normal.

Investigations show:

Hb = 6.4 g/dL
MCV = 131 fl
WBC = 3.1×10^9/L
Platelets = 63×10^9/L

1 *What is the diagnosis?*
2 *Which further investigations are required?*
3 *How would you treat her?*

Case 4

A 64-year-old man is referred for investigation of an elevated haemoglobin concentration (Hb = 18.9 g/dL). He had been well until 4 months previously when he had developed weakness of his right arm and leg. This was confirmed by CT scan to be due to a thrombosis of the left middle cerebral artery. He had given up smoking 2 years ago. He gave a history of intermittent chest pain thought to be related to angina.

On examination, he is overweight (89 kg). His blood pressure is normal (130/80). His pulse was regular and examination of chest is normal. On examination of his abdomen, it was difficult to be certain whether or not he had enlarged and palpable spleen. The area of splenic dullness appeared to be increased.

Investigations show:

Hb = 18.9 g/dL
WBC = 12.3×10^9/L
Neutrophils = 9.7×10^9/L (raised)
MCV = 72
Platelets = 634×10^9/L
Urea and electrolytes – normal
Liver function tests – normal
ECG – normal
Cardiac rhythm – normal.

1 *What is the differential diagnosis of the elevated haemoglobin concentration?*
2 *What further tests would you do to establish the cause?*
3 *What treatment would you recommend?*

Case 5

A 55-year-old male is referred for investigation of an enlarged spleen. He attended his GP because of discomfort in the left upper abdomen, and his GP found him to have a palpably enlarged spleen. He is otherwise well and asymptomatic. The GP performed a full blood count, which showed the following results:

Hb = 11.1 g/dL
WBC = 3.2×10^9/L
White cell differential – normal
Platelets = 95×10^9/L

1 *What special features in the history will you enquire about?*
2 *What is the differential diagnosis?*
3 *What further tests will you undertake?*

Case 6

A 56-year-old lady has a blood test performed to check her cholesterol level. The full blood count was found to be abnormal as follows:

Hb = 14.7 g/dL
White cells = 7.6×10^9/L
Platelets = 43×10^9/L

She is well and asymptomatic.

Physical examination was undertaken. She has occasional bruises over her legs, but no other abnormality is detected.

1 *What is the differential diagnosis?*
2 *What further specific questions would you ask in the history?*
3 *What tests would you do?*
4 *How would you treat her?*

Case 7

A 27-year-old male developed pain in his right calf associated with swelling of the foot. He had recently returned from New Zealand and had undertaken a 12-hour flight from Singapore to London. He was a non-smoker. He was otherwise in generally very good health.

On specific questioning, he revealed that his mother and father were well, although his father had suffered deep vein thrombosis on two occasions. He had two brothers and a sister and his sister had suffered a deep vein thrombosis soon after starting treatment with the contraceptive pill.

He was not on any medication.

1 *What is the likely diagnosis?*
2 *What other tests would you perform?*
3 *What treatment would you undertake?*

Case 8

A 31-year-old lady delivers a healthy male child of 40 weeks gestation. First stage of labour is normal; however, soon after delivery, the patient experiences a substantial blood loss. She becomes hypotensive. An urgent full blood count showed the following:

Hb = 6.7 g/dL
White cells = 14.7×10^9/L – differential normal
Platelets = 67×10^9/L.

1 *What aspects of immediate management are important?*
2 *What other treatments would you institute?*

Case 9

A 73-year-old lady develops shingles (herpes zoster infection) in the right T7 dermatome. She attends her GP who also notices that she has palpable lymph nodes in the right cervical region. The general practitioner undertakes a full blood count, which shows the following:

Hb = 13.1 g/dL
White cells = 27.7×10^9/L
Lymphocytes = 82%
Platelets = 277×10^9/L
Blood film – predominance of mature lymphoid cells

1 *What is the likely diagnosis?*
2 *What further tests would you undertake?*
3 *What treatment would you institute?*

Case 10

A 22-year-old man is noted to have a swelling in the right supraclavicular region. He has complained of cough some 3 months ago and was diagnosed to have a chest infection which was appropriately treated with antibiotics. He has noticed 3 kg of weight loss over the past 6 months. He has otherwise been in generally good health. There is no other relevant history. He is a non-smoker.

On examination, he has a palpable lymph node in the right supraclavicular region measuring 1.5 cm. He has multiple scratch marks over his upper thorax and back and gives a history of pruritus.

1 *What is the differential diagnosis?*
2 *How would you manage this patient?*

Answers to MCQs

1 (a) False. MCV is usually low.
  (b) True.
  (c) False. Is most commonly due to bleeding.
  (d) True.
  (e) False. The rate of response is similar and related to time taken for haemopoiesis to occur (5–7 days).

2 (a) False. Renal failure is usually associated with a normochromic normocytic anaemia.
  (b) True, e.g. pernicious anaemia, vegetarianism, post-gastrectomy.
  (c) False. The anaemia of chronic disease is normocytic or mildly microcytic.
  (d) True.
  (e) False.

3 (a) False.
  (b) False. Bone marrow failure = anaemia, leucopenia and thrombocytopenia. CML presents with leucocytosis, splenomegaly.
  (c) True. >95% of patients have the Philadelphia chromosome t(9;22).
  (d) True.
  (e) True.

4 (a) True.
  (b) False.
  (c) False. Median survival is 7–10 years.
  (d) True. Up to 30% of patients.
  (e) True. >95% are B cells.

5 (a) True.
  (b) False.
  (c) True.
  (d) True.
  (e) False. Monocytes often raised >1000 × 10⁹/L (chronic myelomonocytic leukaemia).

6 (a) False. Heparin is preferable during pregnancy. Warfarin is teratogenic.
  (b) False. The INR is used to monitor Warfarin therapy.
  (c) False.
  (d) True. Protamine is used to reverse heparin.
  (e) False. Three months, unless there are any other thrombosis risk factors.

7 (a) False. Factor VIII concentrate or recombinant factor VIII is used.
  (b) False. It is not heat treated. Viral transmission can occur, although the risk is low.
  (c) False. Corticosteroids, immunosuppressives, splenectomy and intravenous γ-globulin.
  (d) True, especially in conjunction with plasma exchange and if first depleted of cryoprecipitate.
  (e) True.

8 (a) True. Due to transplacental passage of maternal IgG antibodies.
  (b) True, e.g. congenital rubella, CMV.
  (c) True, e.g. anti-HPA-1a antibodies.

  (d) True. Due to half-life of maternally derived antibodies.
  (e) True. Thrombocytopenia with absent radii (TAR).

9 (a) False. Anaemia occurs only when marrow compensation fails.
  (b) True.
  (c) False. The anaemia is usually acholuric.
  (d) True. Haemolysis occurs within the marrow and RES.
  (e) True. This is due to deposition of unconjugated bilirubin in the neonatal brain.

10 (a) False. It is commonly seen in parasitic diseases.
  (b) True.
  (c) False. Basophilia is much more common.
  (d) True.
  (e) True.

11 (a) True.
  (b) False. Thalassaemia trait occurs independently of pregnancy.
  (c) True.
  (d) True.
  (e) False. Platelet count often lowered in pregnancy.

12 (a) False. Smokers can develop secondary or spurious polycythaemia.
  (b) True. This is due to hyperuricaemia.
  (c) True. Approximately 5% of cases.
  (d) True. In 2/3 cases.
  (e) True.

13 (a) False. They are a source of thromboxane.
  (b) False. They do not have nuclei.
  (c) True.
  (d) True.
  (e) True.

14 (a) False.
  (b) True.
  (c) True.
  (d) False.
  (e) True.

15 (a) False. It is sex-linked.
  (b) False it is autosomal dominant.
  (c) False. There is a 1:4 chance.
  (d) True.
  (e) True.

16 (a) True.
  (b) False.
  (c) False.
  (d) True.
  (e) False.

17 (a) False. Selected, poor risk patients only.
  (b) False. Children generally tolerate the procedure better than adults.
  (c) True.

(d) False. Blood products used in supportive care are irradiated.

(e) False. CMV infection is important, however.

18 (a) False. More commonly B cell.

(b) True.

(c) True.

(d) True.

(e) False. They are increasing.

19 (a) False.

(b) True.

(c) True.

(d) True.

(e) True.

20 (a) False. This is a red cell enzymopathy.

(b) True.

(c) True. As is chronic lymphocytic leukaemia.

(d) False.

(e) False. This is a risk factor for thrombosis.

21 (a) True.

(b) False. The platelet count is usually low.

(c) True.

(d) True.

(e) False. Usually prolonged.

22 (a) False. Reactive proliferations are usually polyclonal.

(b) True.

(c) True.

(d) False.

(e) False. These are found post splenectomy in red cells.

23 (a) False. Heparin activates antithrombin.

(b) True.

(c) False.

(d) False.

(e) False.

24 (a) True.

(b) True.

(c) False.

(d) True.

(e) True.

25 (a) True.

(b) False. Remission rates for ALL and AML >90%.

(c) True.

(d) True.

(e) True.

Answers to case studies

Case 1

A history of anorexia and weight loss suggests occult malignancy. A microcytic anaemia suggests iron deficiency, and the elevated platelet count suggests bleeding as the cause. The raised ESR supports a diagnosis of underlying malignancy.

An accurate dietary and alcohol history should be taken, although alcohol usually causes a macrocytic anaemia. A poor diet may also cause folate or B_{12} deficiency, which would also cause a macrocytic anaemia.

Management: diagnosis and treatment

Further diagnostic tests should include serum ferritin, serum B_{12} and serum folate. Urea and electrolytes and liver function tests should also be done. A search for a cause of bleeding is mandatory, even though physical examination does not offer clues to the source of blood loss. Once iron deficiency is confirmed, endoscopic and/or radiological investigation of the gastrointestinal tract is indicated.

The serum ferritin was reduced at 5 μg/L confirming iron deficiency. Upper gastrointestinal endoscopy revealed a malignant gastric ulcer which was successfully resected.

See Chapter 11 for further details.

Case 2

A history of recent onset of back pain, with poor appetite and weight loss, suggests malignant infiltration of the skeleton. Abdominal pain and constipation are suggestive of hypercalcaemia.

Proteinuria on urine testing suggests renal disease. There is no history of prostatic obstruction. The very high ESR suggests myeloma or carcinoma with bony metastases. Further tests should include urea and electrolytes, creatinine clearance, calcium level and serum alkaline phosphatase. X-rays of his back are required. Serum and urinary protein electrophoresis are needed to exclude myeloma.

A prostate-specific antigen test to exclude prostatic carcinoma is required. This patient's calcium level was raised at 3.6 mmol/L and he was in renal failure (serum creatinine 860 mmol/L).

The serum alkaline phosphatase was normal, which is in keeping with multiple myeloma rather than secondary deposits. Skeletal survey, bone marrow, serum and urine paraprotein level, serum β_2-microglobulin are indicated.

See Chapter 30 for further details.

Case 3

This lady presents a classic clinical picture of pernicious anaemia.

The further investigations required are given in Chapter 14.

Treatment is with hydroxocobalamin (1 mg intramuscular) immediately followed by further B_{12} injections. It is important not to give folic acid before giving B_{12}, as it may precipitate neuropathy.

See Chapter 14 for further details.

Case 4

Differential diagnosis

An elevated haemoglobin concentration and haematocrit can cause an increase in blood viscosity, which can predispose to thrombosis. An elevated haemoglobin concentration may arise because of a genuine increase in red cell mass (true polycythaemia) or a relative increase in red cell mass due, for example, to a reduction in plasma volume (pseudo-polycythaemia). Possible causes of an increased red cell mass in this patient are polycythaemia rubra vera (primary polycythaemia) which is a myeloproliferative condition and secondary polycythaemia due to the elevation of endogenous erythropoietin production. This may arise due to hypoxia consequent upon chronic smoking-induced lung disease. Rarer causes of secondary polycythaemia include a renal cyst or tumour, cyanotic heart disease or an erythropoietin-secreting tumour, e.g. a hepatoma. Possible causes of a reduced plasma volume and pseudo-polycythaemia in this patient include smoking-related 'stress polycythaemia'. However, he is not hypertensive and he is not taking diuretic therapy, which are both common causes of pseudo-polycythaemia. The raised white cell and platelet counts strongly suggest polycythaemia rubra vera.

Further tests

Abdominal ultrasound scan to assess spleen size (raised in polycythaemia rubra vera). This investigation would also exclude renal cysts/tumours. His iron status should be assessed – his low mean cell volume suggests that he may have a low ferritin. Iron deficiency is common in patients with PRV as the excess erythropoietic drive utilizes iron leading to iron deficiency in the presence of a normal or even elevated haemoglobin concentration. His JAK 2 status should be ascertained. More than 95% of patients with polycythaemia rubra vera have a mutation at the JAK 2 locus which serves to disturb signal transduction in the erythropoietic lineage and to increase red cell mass.

Treatment

He should be venesected to maintain a PCV of <0.45. It is important to avoid iron which can accelerate erythropoiesis and lead to uncontrolled polycythaemia. He should receive low-dose aspirin thromboprophylaxis. Chemotherapy, e.g. oral hydroxyurea can be considered if venesection alone is insufficient to maintain his haemoglobin in the correct range. Treatment of secondary polycythaemia is much more difficult and should be directed at the cause. This patient was found to have a heterozygous mutation at the JAK II locus and a diagnosis of true polycythaemia rubra vera was made. Strictly speaking, there is no reason to perform a bone marrow aspirate and trephine biopsy in this setting; however, if a trephine biopsy were performed, it would demonstrate increased cellularity of the marrow often with an increase in fibrosis.

See Chapter 27 for further details.

Case 5
Special features
The following specific features should be covered in the history. Alcohol consumption can lead to chronic liver disease, which is a common cause of splenomegaly. Acute alcohol consumption can also lead to acute liver disease which in this setting can also cause an enlarged spleen. Any history of liver disease, e.g. jaundice, recent travel, a detailed drug history and any history of bleeding, e.g. from varices or piles, will be relevant. Evidence of bone marrow failure revealed in the history as previous infection, bruising, bleeding and symptoms of anaemia should be closely enquired for. A number of infections can cause splenic enlargement and a history of fever, recent travel, enlargement of lymph glands should be taken. Any history of pruritus, fever or weight loss may indicate a haematologic malignancy. Night sweats would be an indicator possibly of haematologic malignancy or of infection. The family history must be closely taken as a number of inherited conditions can present in this way. The patient's past medical history must be taken carefully.

Differential diagnosis
Liver disease – both acute and chronic liver disease with portal hypertension. Haematologic conditions, e.g. malignancies such as lymphoma or hairy cell leukaemia, and less commonly myeloproliferative conditions such as polycythaemia rubra vera or myelofibrosis can present in this way. Other conditions include congestive cardiac failure, infiltrative conditions such as amyloidosis and sarcoidosis and certain immunologic conditions, e.g. Felty's syndrome occurring in rheumatoid arthritis and occasionally connective tissue disorders. Inherited conditions that can present in this way include lysosomal storage diseases, e.g. Gaucher disease, which is particularly common amongst Ashkenazi Jewish individuals. Infections that can cause splenic enlargement include bacterial endocarditis, some viral infections, e.g. infectious mononucleosis, hepatitis viruses, brucellosis, histoplasmosis.

Investigations
Liver function tests, coagulation and other assessment of liver disease including titres for hepatitis viruses and tests for chronic liver disease, e.g. caeruloplasmin, alpha-foetoprotein, serum ferritin to exclude haemochromatosis.

Tests to exclude haematologic malignancy. A careful examination of the blood film is important, e.g. to exclude hairy cell leukaemia, occasionally lymphoma cells may be seen in peripheral blood and a peripheral blood differential must be carefully performed. Flow cytometry of peripheral blood cells can sometimes reveal a minor population of lymphoma cells.

A CT scan or other imaging of the abdomen should be undertaken to carefully assess spleen size, liver size and texture and look for other intra-abdominal pathology, e.g. lymphadenopathy. A bone marrow aspirate and trephine biopsy should be undertaken to look for infiltrative conditions. A monospot can be done to look for infectious mononucleosis, other tests for infections should be undertaken depending on the clinical circumstances, e.g. peripheral blood screening for presence of malaria parasites.

See Chapter 5 for further details.

Case 6
Differential diagnosis
The differential diagnosis of a low platelet count includes causes of reduced platelet production by the bone marrow and causes of increased platelet destruction or sequestration of platelets. Sequestration of platelets usually occurs in the spleen and it is noteworthy that the spleen is not palpable. Sequestration can occasionally occur within a giant haemangioma, but no specific skin abnormalities have been noted in this patient.

Reduced platelet production can arise due to infiltration of the bone marrow. This would usually lead to a reduction in red cells and white cells or abnormalities of these cells in addition to thrombocytopenia. Aplastic anaemia or drug-induced bone marrow damage is also likely to cause pancytopenia. This has not been observed in this patient, suggesting that reduced production is unlikely.

Increased destruction of platelets most frequently occurs due to antibody-mediated destruction of platelets. Accelerated consumption of platelets can occur in the setting of coagulation abnormalities, e.g. disseminated intravascular coagulation (DIC) wherein platelets are consumed as part of a coagulopathy or in thrombotic thrombocytopenic purpura (TTP). This patient is generally well and this would make DIC or TTP unlikely, as these conditions are usually seen in severely ill patients, often with other organ damage, e.g. renal failure.

Another common cause of mild thrombocytopenia such as this is spurious thrombocytopenia due to platelet clumping. The blood cell count must be repeated. The platelet clumping sometimes particularly occurs in EDTA samples and a platelet count from citrated blood should also be undertaken. The clumps of platelets will be visible on the peripheral blood film. Specific further history that must be taken includes a very careful history of drugs as various drugs can cause thrombocytopenia. A history of bleeding or bruising should be taken in any patient with thrombocytopenia. Any history of connective tissue disorder affecting skin or joints might be a clue to a generalized immune disturbance. The spleen is not palpable but it could be two to three times enlarged before it becomes palpable. A history of liver disease or of any condition that may increase spleen size should also be undertaken.

Further tests
It is important to repeat the blood count. Screening for connective tissue disturbances including an anti-nuclear factor and rheumatoid factor should be undertaken. Assessment of platelet antibodies can be undertaken, but these tests are usually difficult to perform and often give non-specific results.

Bone marrow aspirate and trephine biopsy should be considered to assess platelet production.

An abdominal CT scan should be considered to assess spleen size and exclude other intra-abdominal pathology, e.g. lymphadenopathy.

Viral titres should be undertaken.

The final diagnosis in this particular patient was mild immune thrombocytopenia. She did not require treatment – it is unusual to develop significant bleeding when the platelet count is above 20×10^9/L.

Treatment

Treatment in patients such as this should be directed towards the cause.

See Chapter 37 for further details.

Case 7
Likely diagnosis

Deep vein thrombosis in the right calf. This should be confirmed by use of appropriate ultrasound and Doppler studies.

Further testing

The family history suggests that there may be an inherited tendency towards thrombophilia and a thrombophilia screen should be conducted. Specific conditions that must be excluded include the presence of factor V Leiden, anti-thrombin deficiency, prothrombin mutations, protein C and protein S deficiency. This patient was found to be heterozygous for factor V Leiden. Activated factor V Leiden is relatively resistant to inactivation by protein C. The risk of thrombosis is increased by 5–10-fold in heterozygotes and 50–100-fold in homozygotes. Up to 5% of the Northern European population are heterozygous for this mutation.

Treatment

He should receive anticoagulation with warfarin with a target INR ratio of 2.0–3.0. Anticoagulation should be continued for a minimum period of 6 months. Long-term prophylactic anticoagulation is probably not indicated but the patient should be warned that he is at risk of recurrent thrombosis. Every effort must be taken to reduce other risk factors for thrombosis, e.g. smoking, being overweight, taking particular care at times of haemostasis, e.g. prophylaxis with heparin prior to a intercontinental flight.

See Chapter 40 for further details.

Case 8
Management

A coagulation profile must be obtained in this patient. There was evidence of DIC (prothrombin time 18 seconds and APTT 54 seconds – both prolonged), thrombin time 21 seconds (prolonged), fibrinogen 0.1 g/L (reduced), fibrin degradation products (FDP) markedly elevated. Immediate transfusion of blood component must be undertaken and all efforts taken to maintain the blood pressure. Crystalloid infusions should be commenced whilst awaiting blood. O-negative blood can be given urgently and compatible red cells must be transfused as soon as available.

Efforts must be taken to establish the cause of disseminated intravascular coagulation. In this setting, it could be due to retained products of conception; the obstetrician may wish to organize an appropriate examination under anaesthetic with evacuation of these retained products. Intravenous antibiotic therapy should be administered.

Other treatments

Further transfusion support should be administered. This would include infusion of fresh frozen plasma and platelets in order to replace consumed coagulation factors and platelets. Cryoprecipitate is a rich source of coagulation factors. Regular monitoring of full blood count, platelet count and coagulation parameters must be instituted. If bleeding persists despite replacement of platelets and clotting factors and cryoprecipitate, recombinant human factor VIIa should be considered. Other treatments that are of value in DIC include infusions of recombinant protein C and infusions of anti-thrombin.

See Chapter 39 for further details.

Case 9
Likely diagnosis

This patient presents with a lymphocytosis of mature cells. The likely diagnosis is chronic lymphocytic leukaemia. This patient would have been a Binet stage A. She has an infection and is immunosuppressed. She should be treated with antiviral treatment, e.g. aciclovir.

Further tests

Flow cytometry of peripheral blood lymphocytes should be undertaken. In CLL, the malignant cells are positive for the CD19 and 22 antigens and are also CD5 positive. The cells will be clonal, i.e. they will express only kappa or lambda light chains. Serum levels of immunoglobulins are typically depressed in chronic lymphocytic leukaemia leading to generalized immune suppression. The expression of ZAP70 should be assessed – ZAP70 positive and CD38 positive CLL has a poor prognosis. The degree of somatic mutation in the immunoglobulin heavy chain genes relates to prognosis – mutated genes generally indicate a favourable prognosis, whereas unmutated genes indicate a more primitive cell and are usually associated with a worse prognosis. Cytogenetic analysis should also be undertaken.

Treatment

This patient should be treated with aciclovir. Treatment of chronic lymphocytic leukaemia Binet stage A is with observation only. There is no evidence that institution of chemotherapy at this stage will be of benefit. This patient should be closely followed.

See Chapter 39 for further details.

Case 10
Differential diagnosis

This gentleman has a significantly enlarged lymph node and requires biopsy. There is no local explanation for the lymphadenopathy. Biopsy showed the appearances of nodular sclerosing Hodgkin's disease.

Further investigation must include accurate staging of the tumour. In addition to clinical evaluation, he should undergo CT scan of chest and abdomen to look for lymphadenopathy and to assess whether or not other non-lymphoid organs are infiltrated. He should also undergo bone marrow aspirate and trephine biopsy. A PET scan can also be undertaken at presentation. In the current case, his CT scan showed extensive intra-abdominal and intra-thoracic lymphadenopathy with evidence of infiltration of the lungs. PET scan confirmed widespread lymphadenopathy and active uptake was demonstrated in lung and liver. He therefore has stage 4B Hodgkin's disease.

He was treated with combination chemotherapy in the form of ABVD (adriamycin, bleomycin, vinblastin, dacarbazine).

Sperm cryopreservation was undertaken prior to commencement of chemotherapy. It would be customary to repeat the PET scan after two courses and to change to more intensive therapy if the scan remained positive, but to continue with six cycles of ABVD if the scan was negative.

See Chapter 31 for further details.

Appendix I: Glossary

Anaemia: a haemoglobin concentration in peripheral blood below normal range for sex and age.

Anisocytosis: variation in size of peripheral blood red cells.

Basophil: a mature circulating white cell with dark purple-staining cytoplasmic granules which may obscure the nucleus.

Chromatin: nuclear material containing DNA and protein.

Clone: a group of cells all derived by mitotic division from a single somatic cell.

Eosinophil: mature circulating white cell with multiple orange-staining cytoplasmic granules and two or three nuclear lobes.

Fluorescent in situ hybridisation (FISH): the use of fluorescently labelled DNA probes which hybridise to chromosomes or sub-chromosomal sequences to detect chromosome deletions or translocations.

Haematocrit: the proportion of a sample of blood taken up by red cells.

Haemoglobin: the red protein in red cells which is composed of four globin chains each containing an iron-containing haem group.

Karyotype: the chromosomal make-up of a cell.

Leukocytosis: a rise in white cell levels in the peripheral blood to above the normal range.

Leukopenia: a fall in white cell (leukocyte) levels in the peripheral blood to below the normal range.

Lymphocyte: a white cell with a single, usually round, nucleus and scanty dark blue-staining cytoplasm. Lymphocytes divide into two main groups: B cells, which produce immunoglobulins; and T cells, which are involved in graft rejection and immunity against viruses.

Macrocytic: red cells of average volume (MCV) above normal.

Mean cell volume (MCV): the average volume of circulating red cells.

Mean corpuscular haemoglobin (MCH): the average haemoglobin content of red blood cells.

Megaloblastic: an abnormal appearance of nucleated red cells in which the nuclear chromatin remains open and fine despite maturation of the cytoplasm.

Microcytic: red cells of average volume (MCV) below normal.

Monocyte: mature circulating white cell with a few pink- or blue-staining cytoplasmic granules, pale blue cytoplasm and a single nucleus. There are usually cytoplasmic vacuoles. In the tissues, the monocyte becomes a macrophage.

Myeloblast: an early granulocyte precursor containing nucleoli and with a primitive nucleus; there may be some cytoplasmic granules.

Myelocyte: a later granulocyte precursor containing granules, a single lobed nucleus and semi-condensed chromatin.

Neutrophil: a mature white cell containing two to five nuclear lobes and many reddish or purple cytoplasmic granules.

Normoblast: (erythroblast): nucleated red cell precursor normally found only in bone marrow.

Pancytopenia: a fall in peripheral blood red cell, white cell and platelet levels to below normal.

Pappenheimer body: an iron granule in red cells stained by standard (Romanovsky) stain.

Paraprotein: a γ-globulin band on protein electrophoresis consisting of identical molecules derived from a clone of plasma cells.

PET scan: positron emission tomography scan used to detect the sites of active disease, e.g. lymphoma.

Phagocyte: a white blood cell that engulfs bacteria or dead tissue. It includes neutrophils and monocytes (macrophages).

Plasma cell: usually an oval-shaped cell, derived from a B lymphocyte, which secretes immunoglobulin. Plasma cells are found in normal bone marrow but not in normal peripheral blood.

Platelet: the smallest cell in peripheral blood, it is non-nucleated and involved in promoting haemostasis.

Poikilocytosis: variation in shape of peripheral blood red cells.

Polycythaemia: a haemoglobin concentration in peripheral blood above normal range for age and sex.

Red cell: mature non-nucleated cell carrying haemoglobin. The most abundant cell in peripheral blood.

Reticulocyte: a non-nucleated young red cell still containing RNA and found in peripheral blood.

Sideroblast: a nucleated red cell precursor found in marrow and containing iron granules, which appear blue with Perls' stain

Siderocyte: a mature red cell containing iron granules and found in peripheral blood or marrow.

Stem cell: resides in the bone marrow and by division and differentiation gives rise to all the blood cells. The stem cell also reproduces itself. Some stem cells circulate in the peripheral blood.

Thrombocytopenia: a platelet level in peripheral blood below the normal range.

Thrombocytosis: a platelet level in peripheral blood above the normal range.

Tissue factor: a protein on the surface of cells which initiates blood coagulation.

White cell (leukocyte): nucleated cell that circulates in peripheral blood and whose main function is combating infections. White cells include granulocytes (neutrophils, eosinophils, and basophils), monocytes and lymphocytes.

von Willebrand factor: a plasma protein that carries factor VIII and mediates the adhesion of platelets to the vessel wall.

Appendix II: Normal values

Normal peripheral blood count

Cell	Normal concentration
Haemoglobin	11.5–15.5 (female)
	13.5–17.5 (male)
Red cell	$3.9–5.6 \times 10^{12}$/L (female)
	$4.5–6.5 \times 10^{12}$/L (male)
Reticulocyte	0.5–3.5%
	$\sim 25–95 \times 10^9$/L
White cells	$4.0–11.0 \times 10^9$/L
Neutrophils	$2.5–7.5 \times 10^3$/L
	($1.5–7.5 \times 10^9$/L in black people)
Eosinophils	$0.04–0.4 \times 10^9$/L
Basophils	$0.01–0.1 \times 10^9$/L
Monocytes	$0.2–0.8 \times 10^9$/L
Lymphocytes	$1.5–3.0 \times 10^9$/L
Haematocrit	0.38–0.54
Mean cell volume	80–100
Mean cell haemoglobin	27–33
Haematinics	
Serum iron	10–30 μmol/L
Total iron binding capacity	40–75 μmol/L (2–4 g/L as transferrin)
Serum ferritin	40–340 μg/L (males)
	15–150 μg/L (females)
Serum folate	3.0–15.0 μg/L (4–30 nmol/L)
Red cell folate	160–640 μg/L (360–1460 nmol/L)
Serum vitamin B_{12}	160–925 μg/L (120–682 pmol/L)

Appendix III: Cluster of differentiation nomenclature system

Cell surface markers are molecules in the cell membrane that can be recognized by reactivity with specific monoclonal antibodies. Their presence gives information about the lineage, function or stage of development of a particular cell population. The cluster of differentiation (CD) nomenclature system groups together antibodies recognizing the same surface molecule (antigen).

T-cell markers	Remarks
CD number	
1a, b, c	Thymocytes, Langerhans' cells (CD1a)
2	E-rosette receptor. All T cells
3	T-cell receptor. Mature T cells
4	T helper/inducer subset
5	T cells (aberrantly expressed in B-CLL, mantle cell lymphoma)
7	T cells (aberrantly expressed in some AML)
8	T cytotoxic/suppressor

B-cell markers	
CD number	
19	B cells, including early B cells
20	Mature B cells
21	Mature B cells. C3d receptor, EBV receptor
22	B cells
23	Activated B cells
79	B cell antigen receptor
103	Hairy cells
138	Plasma cells

Myeloid and other markers
Myeloid markers

CD number	
11a, 11b, 11c	Adhesion molecule ligand. Also expressed on some B and T cells and monocytes
13	All mature myeloid cells
33	Myelin-associated protein. Early myeloid cells
61	Early myeloid cells
117	Early myeloid cells

Others

CD number	
14	Monocytes, macrophages
25	IL-2 receptor-activated B cells
34	Stem cells
45	Leucocyte common antigen: all haemopoietic cells
56	Natural killer cells
9, 29, 31, 41, 42	Platelet markers
38	Plasma cell marker
71	Red cell precursors
TdT	Terminal deoxynucleotidyl transferase – early B- and T-cell precursors

Appendix IV: Further reading

Arceci RJ, Hann IM, Smith OP (eds) (2006) *Pediatric Hematology* (3rd edn). Blackwell Publishing, Oxford.

Hoffbrand AV, Moss PAH, Pettit JE (2006) *Essential Haematology* (5th edn). Wiley-Blackwell, Oxford.

Hoffbrand AV, Catovsky D, Tuddenham EGD (eds) (2005) *Postgraduate Haematology* (5th edn). Blackwell Publishing, Oxford

Hoffman R, Benz EJ, Shattil SJ, Furie B, Cohen HJ, Silberstein LE, McGlave P (2005) *Hematology: Basic Principles and Practice.* Elsevier Churchill Livingstone, Philadelphia.

Lichtman MA, Beutler E, Kipps TJ, Seligsohn U, Kaushansky K, Prchal JT (2006) *Williams Hematology* (7th edn). McGraw-Hill Medical, New York.

Index

Note: Page numbers in *italic* refer to figures or tables.